This book belongs to:

DENTAL ANATOMY

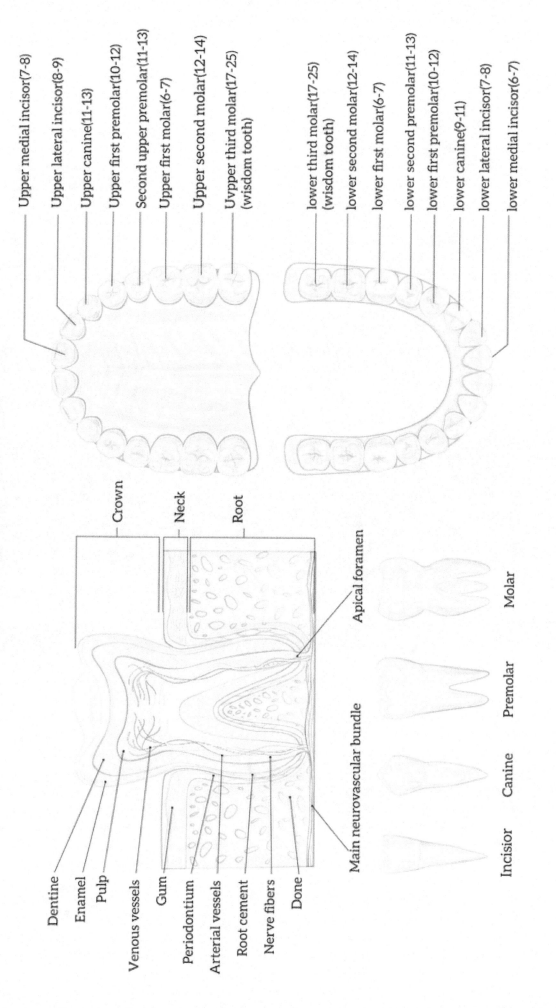

Upper medial incisor(7-8)
Upper lateral incisor(8-9)
Upper canine(11-13)
Upper first premolar(10-12)
Second upper premolar(11-13)
Upper first molar(6-7)
Upper second molar(12-14)
Uvpper third molar(17-25) (wisdom tooth)

lower third molar(17-25) (wisdom tooth)
lower second molar(12-14)
lower first molar(6-7)
lower second premolar(11-13)
lower first premolar(10-12)
lower canine(9-11)
lower lateral incisor(7-8)
lower medial incisor(6-7)

Crown
Neck
Root

Apical foramen
Main neurovascular bundle

Dentine
Enamel
Pulp
Venous vessels
Gum
Periodontium
Arterial vessels
Root cement
Nerve fibers
Done

Incisior   Canine   Premolar   Molar

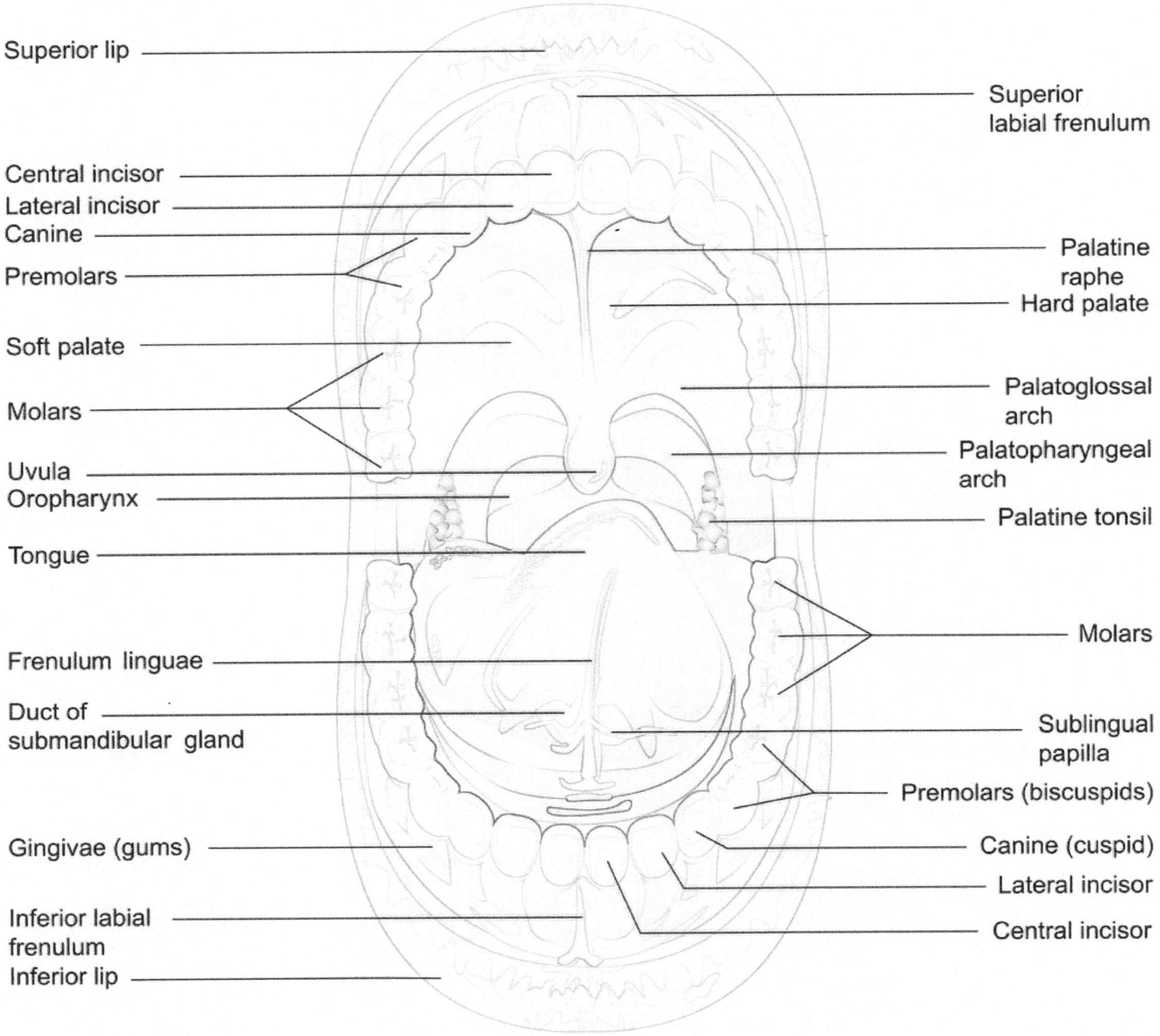

Superior
labial frenulum

Palatine
raphe

Hard palate

Palatoglossal
arch

Palatopharyngeal
arch

Palatine tonsil

Molars

Sublingual
papilla

Premolars (biscuspids)

Canine (cuspid)

Lateral incisor

Central incisor

Superior lip

Central incisor

Lateral incisor

Canine

Premolars

Soft palate

Molars

Uvula

Oropharynx

Tongue

Frenulum linguae

Duct of
submandibular gland

Gingivae (gums)

Inferior labial
frenulum

Inferior lip

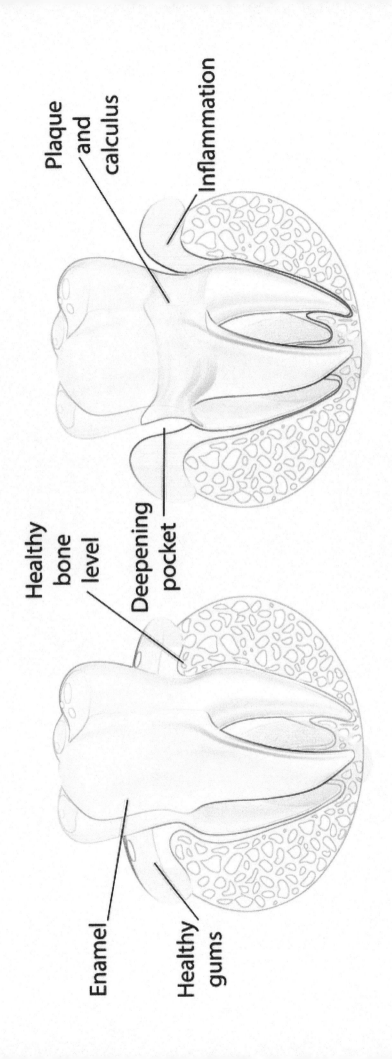

Normal tooth

Periodontitis

Enamel

Healthy gums

Healthy bone level

Deepening pocket

Plaque and calculus

Inflammation

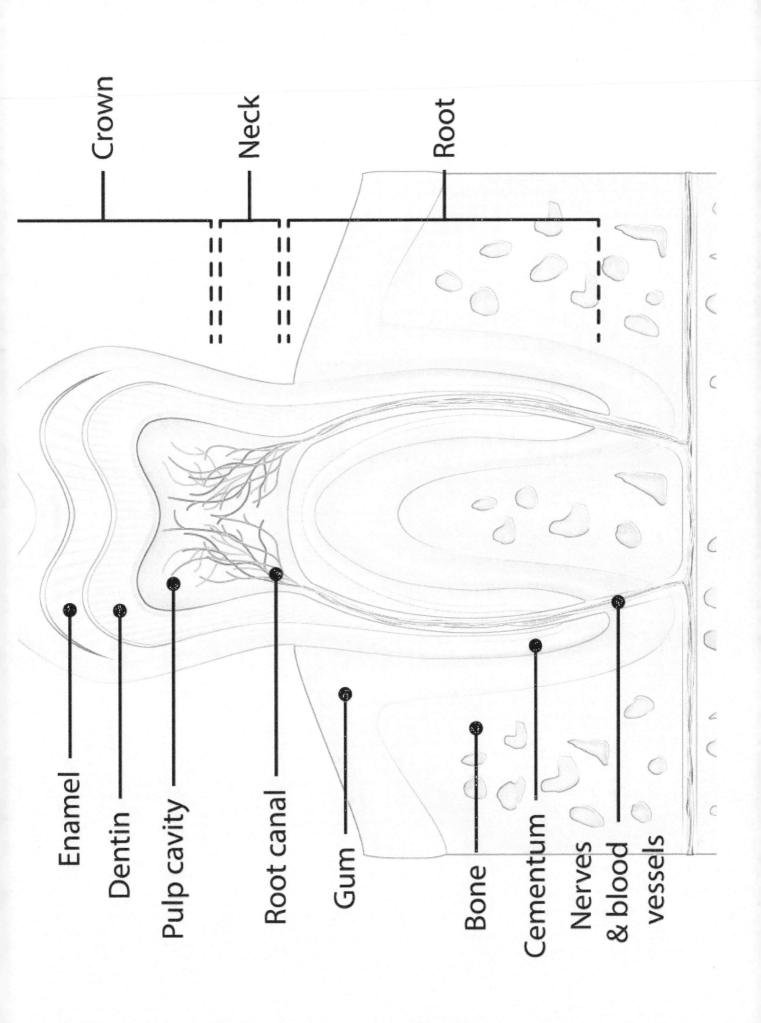

Crown

Neck

Root

Enamel

Dentin

Pulp cavity

Root canal

Gum

Bone

Cementum

Nerves
& blood
vessels

Structure of oral cavity

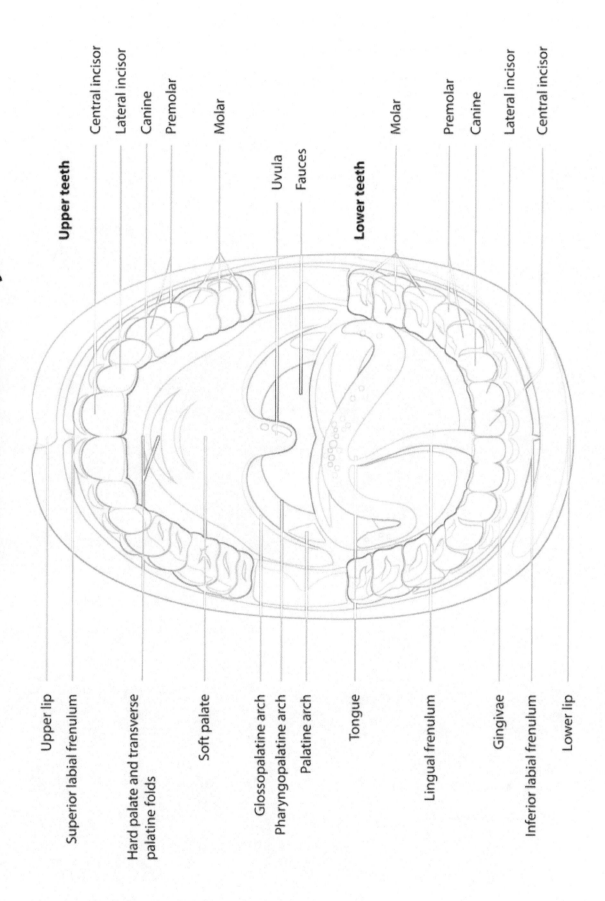

Upper lip

Superior labial frenulum

Hard palate and transverse palatine folds

Soft palate

Glossopalatine arch

Pharyngopalatine arch

Palatine arch

Tongue

Lingual frenulum

Gingivae

Inferior labial frenulum

Lower lip

Upper teeth

Central incisor

Lateral incisor

Canine

Premolar

Molar

Uvula

Fauces

Lower teeth

Molar

Premolar

Canine

Lateral incisor

Central incisor

Tooth Structure

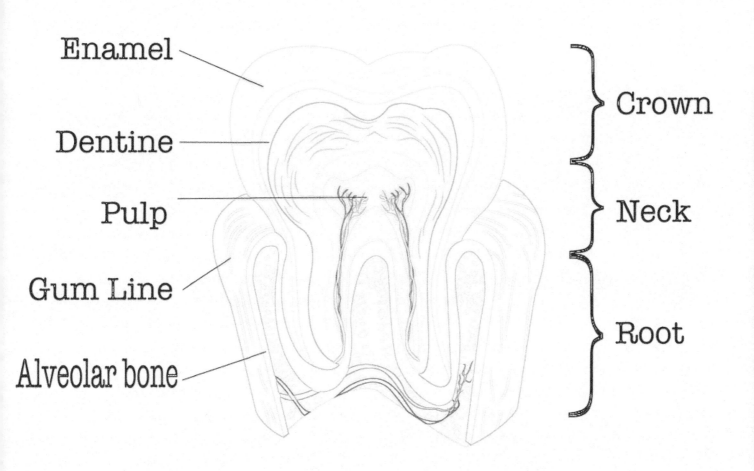

Enamel

Dentine

Pulp

Gum Line

Alveolar bone

Crown

Neck

Root

Root Canal Retreatment

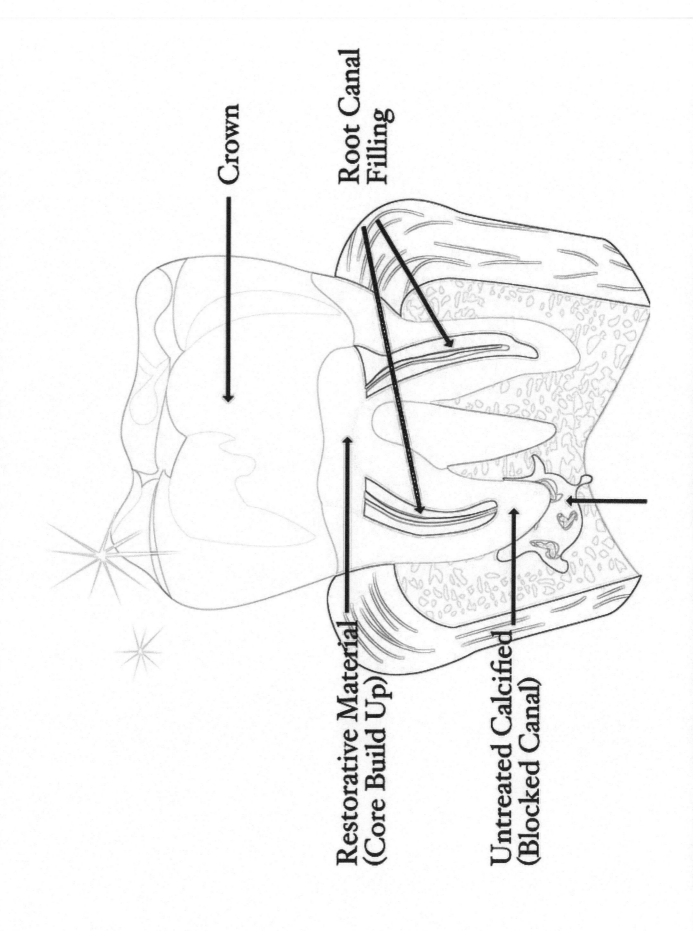

Crown

Root Canal
Filling

Restorative Material
(Core Build Up)

Untreated Calcified
(Blocked Canal)

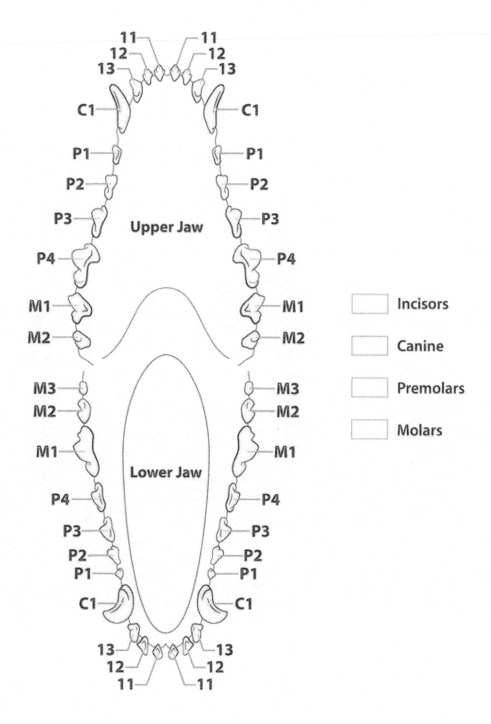

Upper Jaw

Lower Jaw

Incisors

Canine

Premolars

Molars

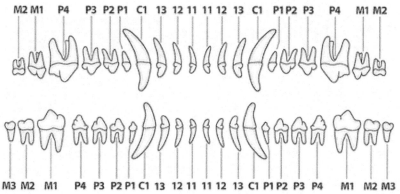

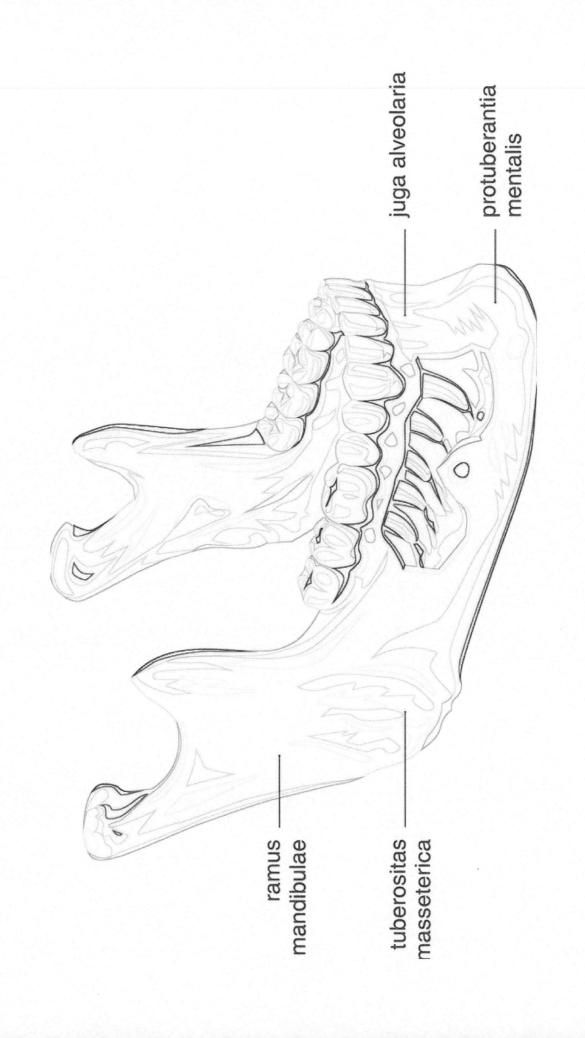

juga alveolaria

protuberantia
mentalis

ramus
mandibulae

tuberositas
masseterica

Enamel Decay

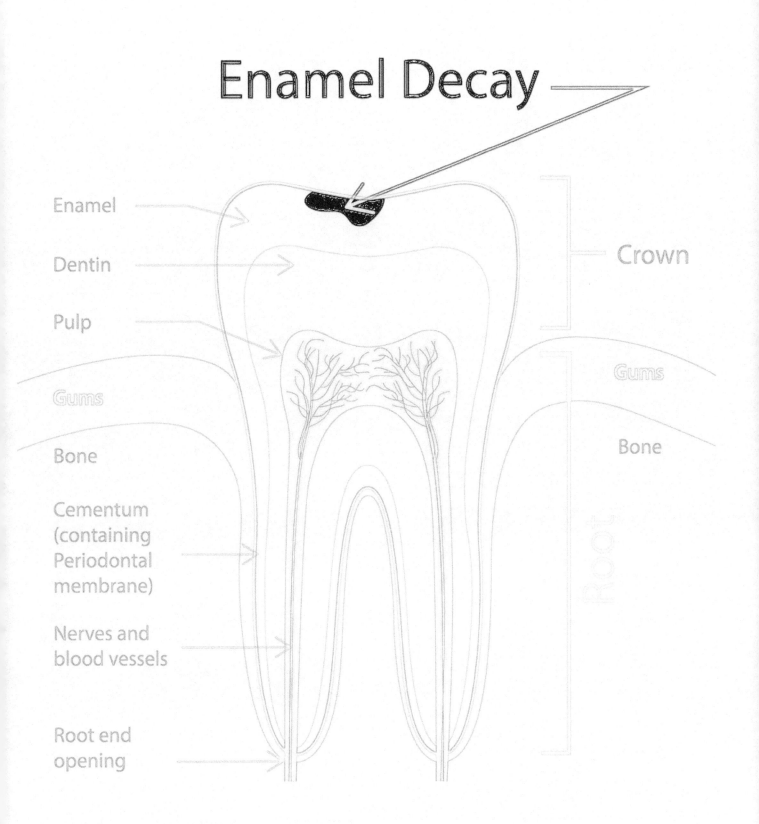

Enamel

Dentin

Pulp

Gums

Bone

Cementum
(containing
Periodontal
membrane)

Nerves and
blood vessels

Root end
opening

Crown

Gums

Bone

Root

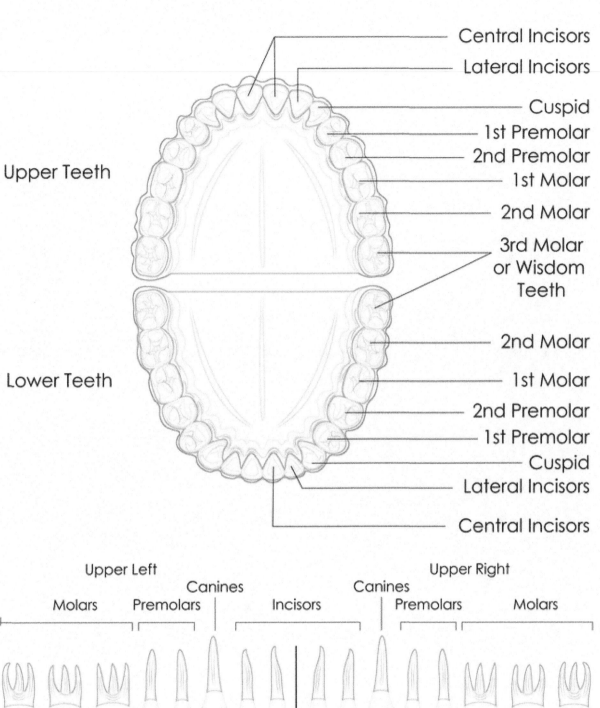

Central Incisors
Lateral Incisors
Cuspid
1st Premolar
2nd Premolar
1st Molar
2nd Molar
3rd Molar or Wisdom Teeth

Upper Teeth

Lower Teeth

2nd Molar
1st Molar
2nd Premolar
1st Premolar
Cuspid
Lateral Incisors
Central Incisors

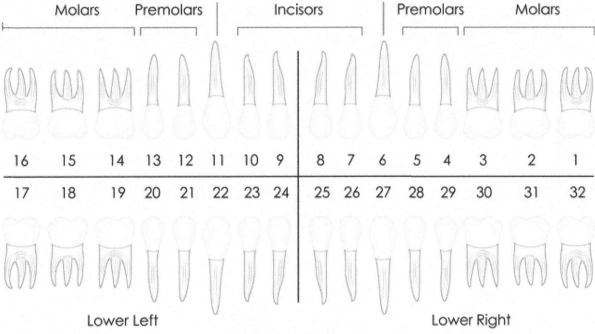

Upper Left								Upper Right							
Molars			Premolars		Canines	Incisors			Canines	Premolars		Molars			
16	15	14	13	12	11	10	9	8	7	6	5	4	3	2	1
17	18	19	20	21	22	23	24	25	26	27	28	29	30	31	32

Lower Left

Lower Right

TEETH

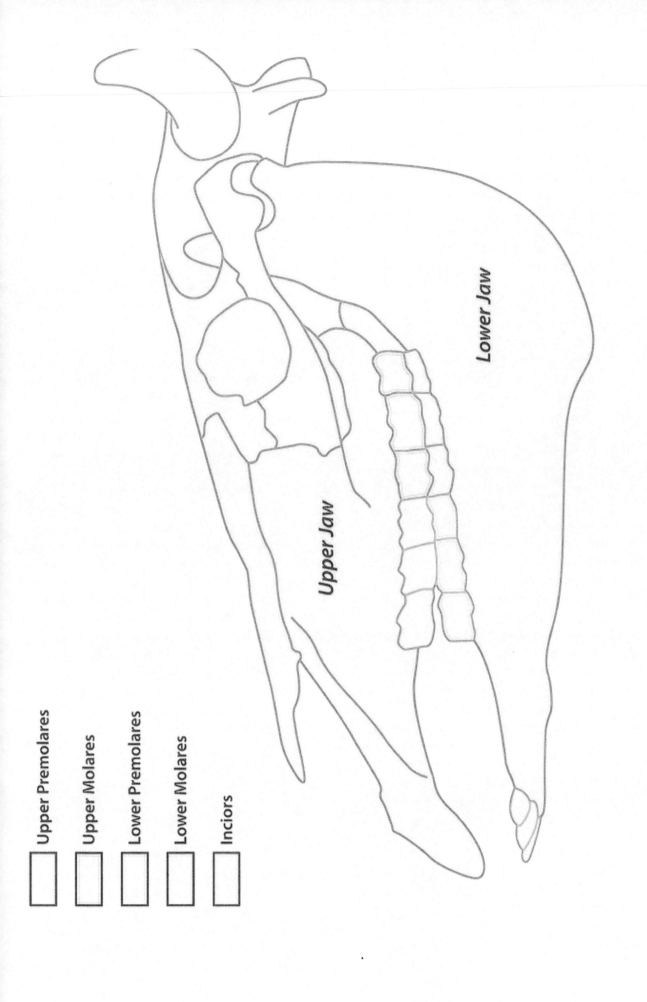

Upper Premolares

Upper Molares

Lower Premolares

Lower Molares

Inciors

Upper Jaw

Lower Jaw

Root Canal Treatment

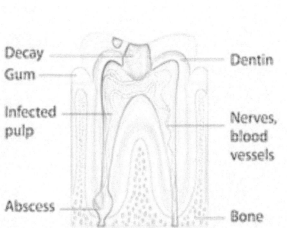

Decay
Gum
Infected pulp
Abscess

Dentin
Nerves, blood vessels
Bone

Infected tooth

Opening

Opening made in tooth

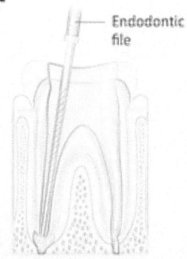

Endodontic file

Infected tissue removed; Canals cleaned

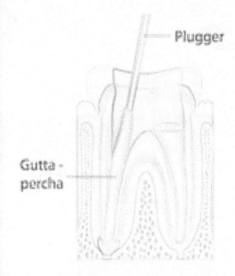

Plugger

Gutta - percha

Canals filled with a permanent material (gutta - percha)

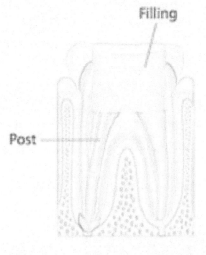

Filling

Post

Opening sealed with filling. In some cases, a post is inserted for extra support

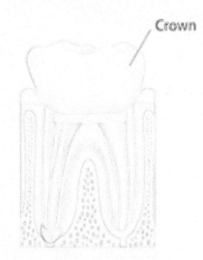

Crown

New crown cemented onto rebuilt tooth

Types of Human Teeth

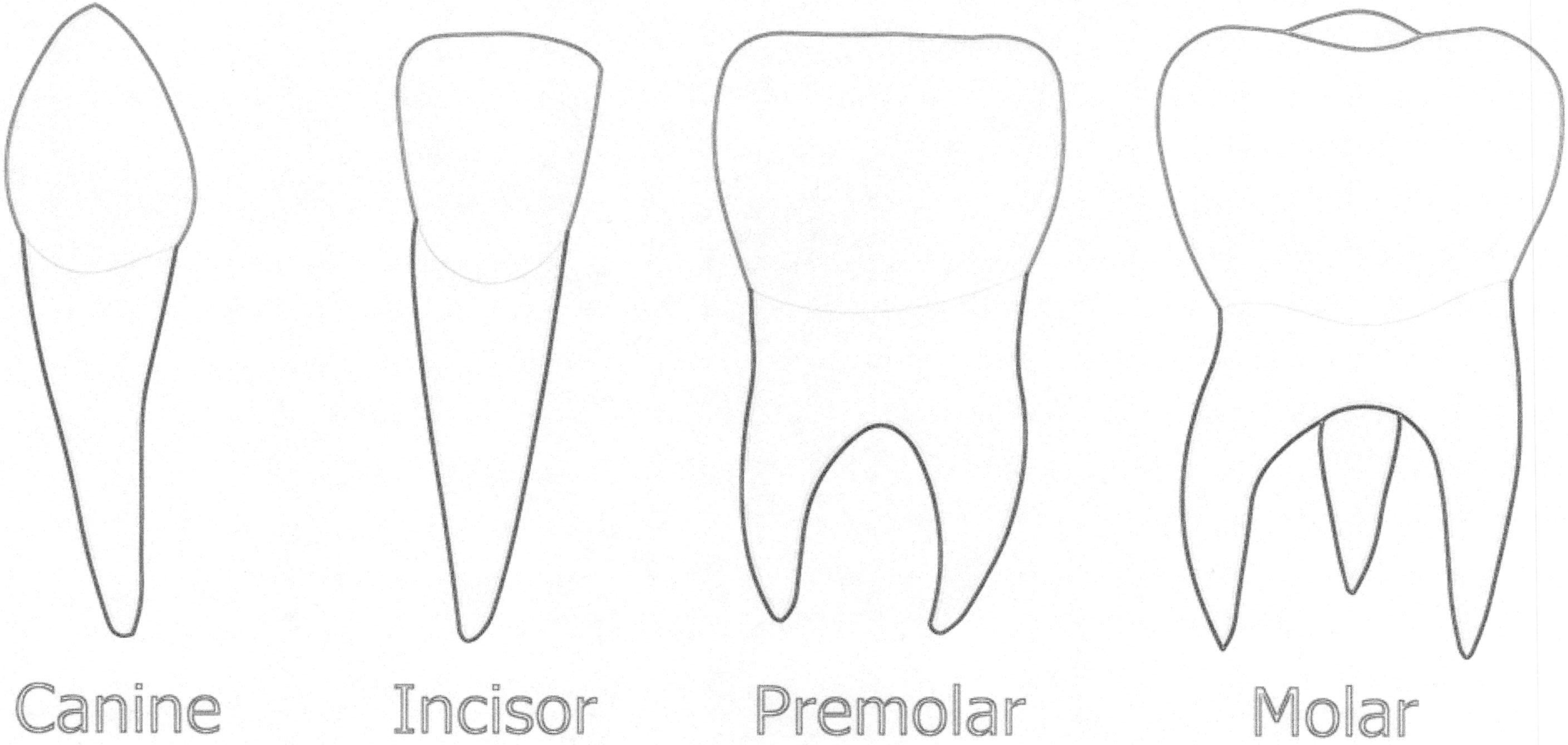

Canine

Incisor

Premolar

Molar

The structure of the tooth

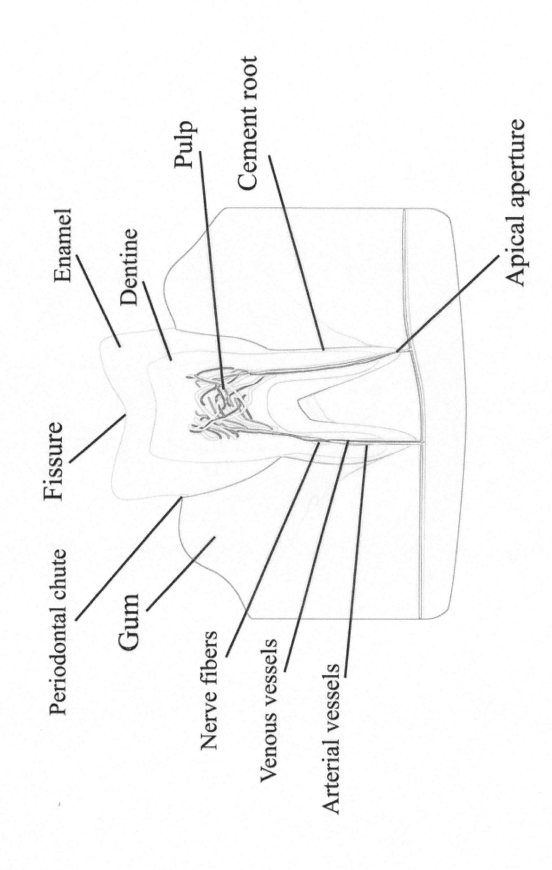

Enamel

Dentine

Pulp

Cement root

Apical aperture

Fissure

Periodontal chute

Gum

Nerve fibers

Venous vessels

Arterial vessels

Shedding (year)

Central incisor (6-7)

Lateral incisor (7-8)

Canine/cuspid (10-12)

First molar (9-11)

Second molar (10-12)

Second molar (10-12)

First molar (9-11)

Canine/cuspid (9-12)

Lateral incisor (7-8)

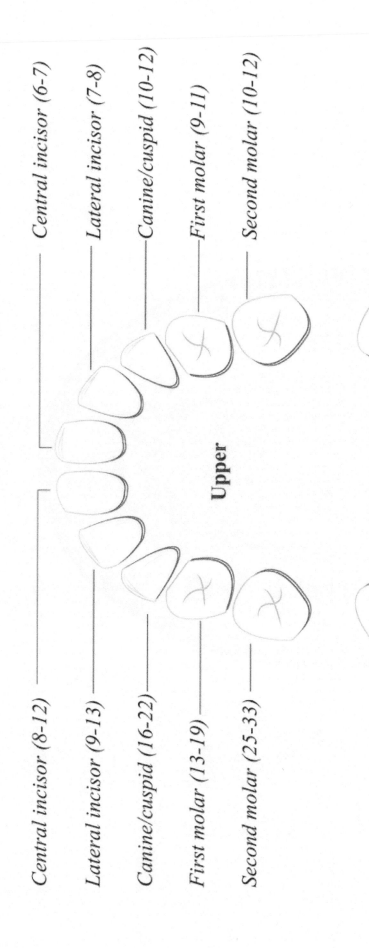

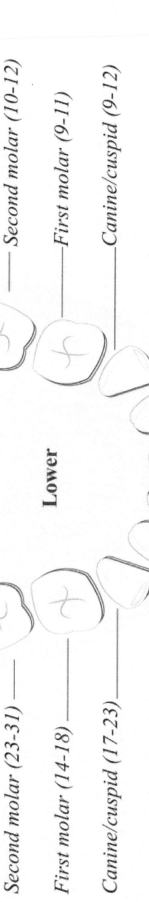

Upper

Lower

Eruption (month)

Central incisor (8-12)

Lateral incisor (9-13)

Canine/cuspid (16-22)

First molar (13-19)

Second molar (25-33)

Second molar (23-31)

First molar (14-18)

Canine/cuspid (17-23)

Lateral incisor (10-16)

Fixed partial denture (bridge)

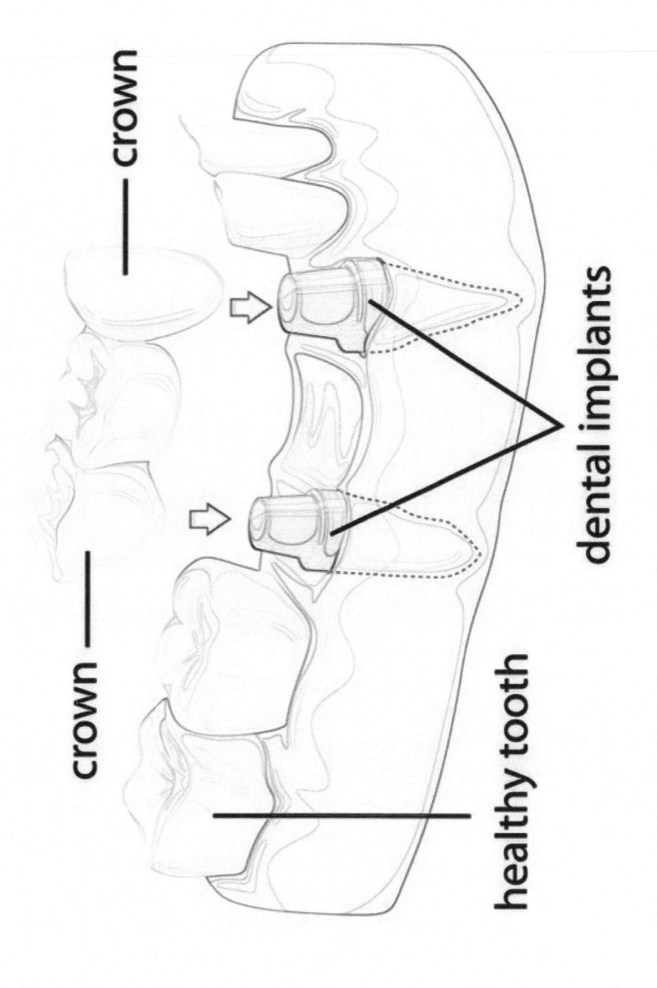

crown

crown

dental implants

healthy tooth

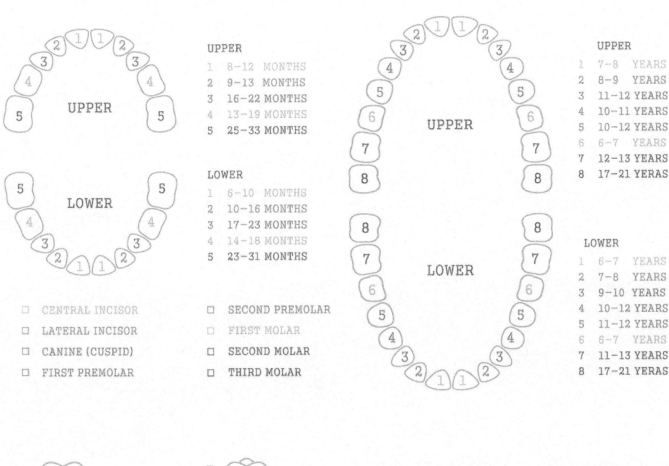

UPPER

1 8-12 MONTHS
2 9-13 MONTHS
3 16-22 MONTHS
4 13-19 MONTHS
5 25-33 MONTHS

LOWER

1 6-10 MONTHS
2 10-16 MONTHS
3 17-23 MONTHS
4 14-18 MONTHS
5 23-31 MONTHS

☐ CENTRAL INCISOR
☐ LATERAL INCISOR
☐ CANINE (CUSPID)
☐ FIRST PREMOLAR

☐ SECOND PREMOLAR
☐ FIRST MOLAR
☐ SECOND MOLAR
☐ THIRD MOLAR

UPPER

1 7-8   YEARS
2 8-9   YEARS
3 11-12 YEARS
4 10-11 YEARS
5 10-12 YEARS
6 6-7   YEARS
7 12-13 YEARS
8 17-21 YERAS

LOWER

1 6-7   YEARS
2 7-8   YEARS
3 9-10 YEARS
4 10-12 YEARS
5 11-12 YEARS
6 6-7   YEARS
7 11-13 YEARS
8 17-21 YERAS

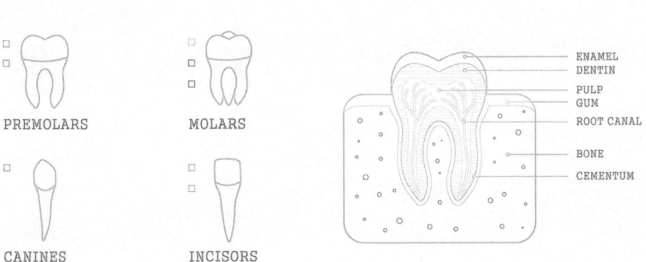

PREMOLARS

MOLARS

CANINES

INCISORS

ENAMEL
DENTIN
PULP
GUM
ROOT CANAL

BONE

CEMENTUM

Tooth Chart

ILLUSTRATION DESIGN

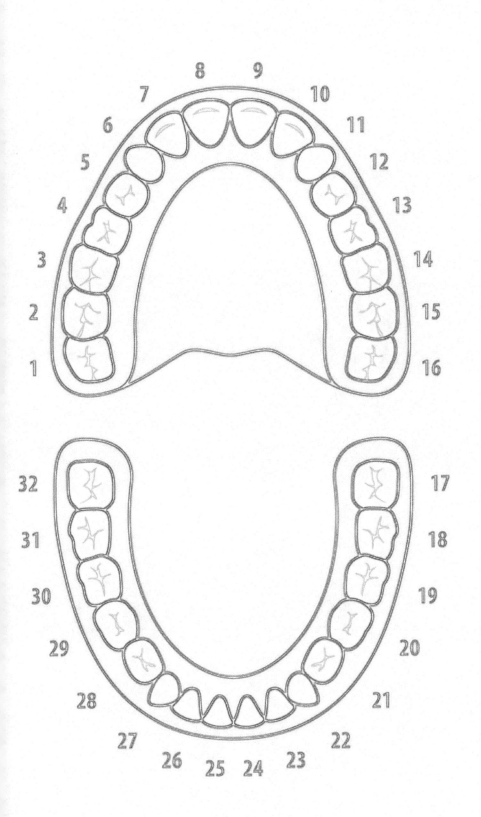

1. 3rd Molar (wisdom tooth)
2. 2nd Molar (12-yr molar)
3. 1st Molar (6-yr molar)
4. 2nd Bicuspid (2nd premolar)
5. 1st Bicuspid (1st premolar)
6. Cuspid (canine/eye tooth)
7. Lateral incisor
8. Central incisor
9. Central incisor
10. Lateral incisor
11. Cuspid (canine/eye tooth)
12. 1st Bicuspid (1st premolar)
13. 2nd Bicuspid (2nd premolar)
14. 1st Molar (6-yr molar)
15. 2nd Molar (12-yr molar)
16. 3rd Molar (wisdom tooth)
17. 3rd Molar (wisdom tooth)
18. 2nd Molar (12-yr molar)
19. 1st Molar (6-yr molar)
20. 2nd Bicuspid (2nd premolar)
21. 1st Bicuspid (1st premolar)
22. Cuspid (canine/eye tooth)
23. Lateral incisor
24. Central incisor
25. Central incisor
26. Lateral incisor
27. Cuspid (canine/eye tooth)
28. 1st Bicuspid (1st premolar)
29. 2nd Bicuspid (2nd premolar)
30. 1st Molar (6-yr molar)
31. 2nd Molar (12-yr molar)
32. 3rd Molar (wisdom tooth)

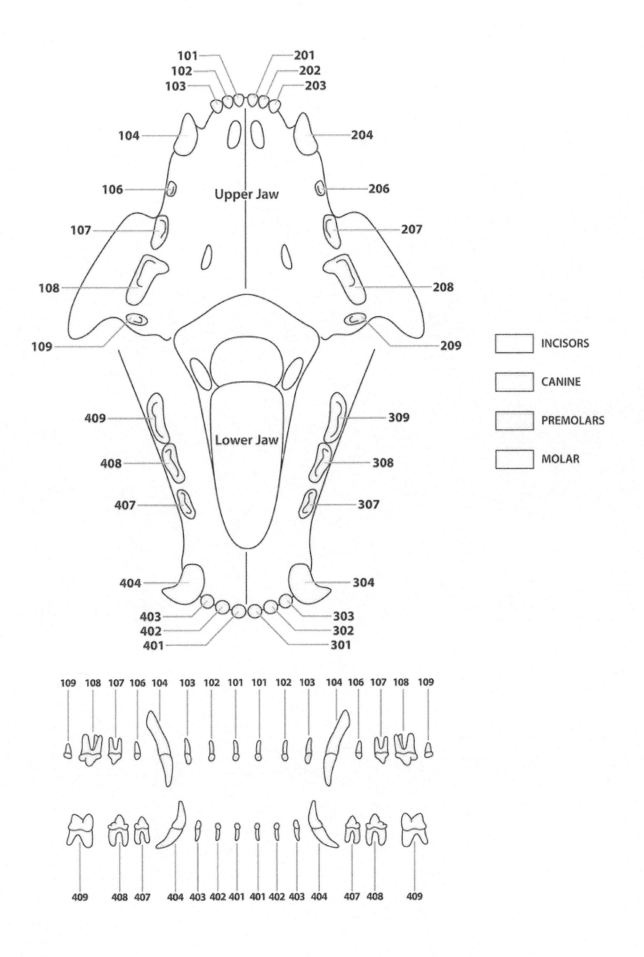

101
102
103
201
202
203
104
204
Upper Jaw
106
206
107
207
108
208
109
209

INCISORS

CANINE

PREMOLARS

MOLAR

409
309
408
308
407
307
Lower Jaw
404
304
403
402
401
303
302
301

109 108 107 106 104 103 102 101 101 102 103 104 106 107 108 109

409 408 407 404 403 402 401 401 402 403 404 407 408 409

Fixed partial denture (bridge)

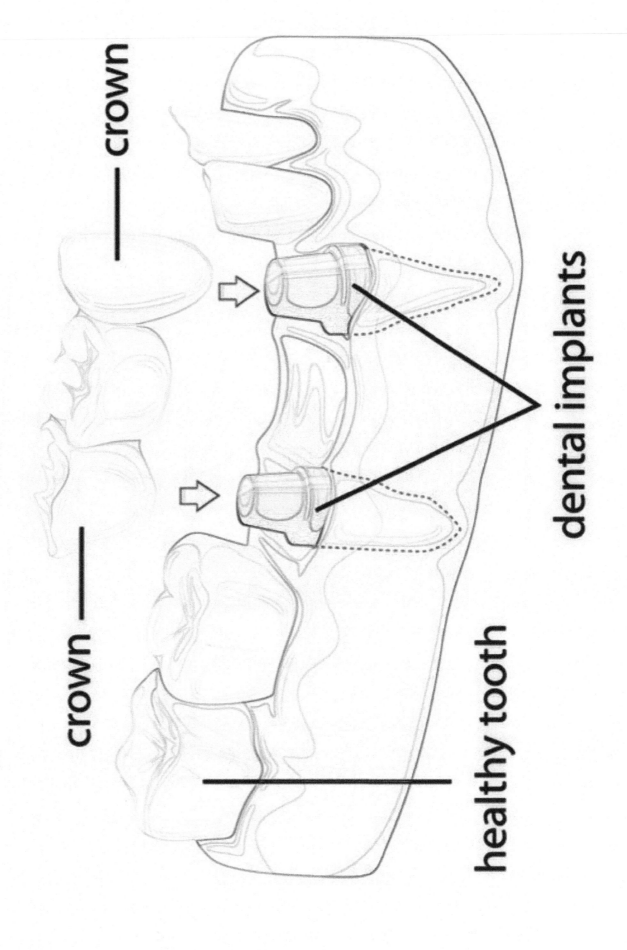

crown

crown

dental implants

healthy tooth

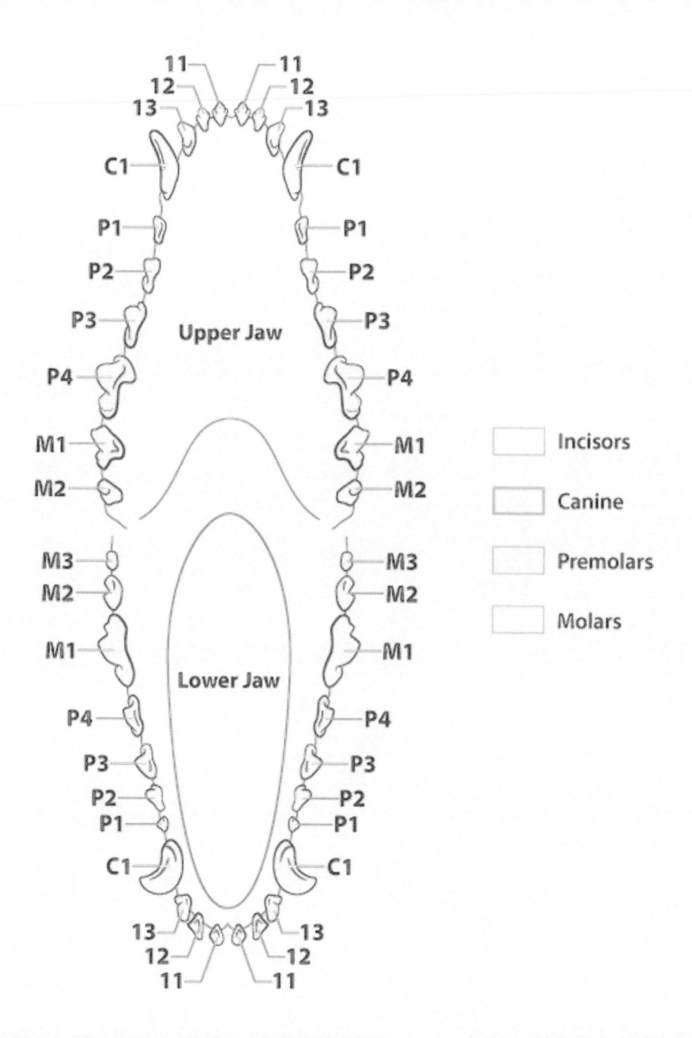

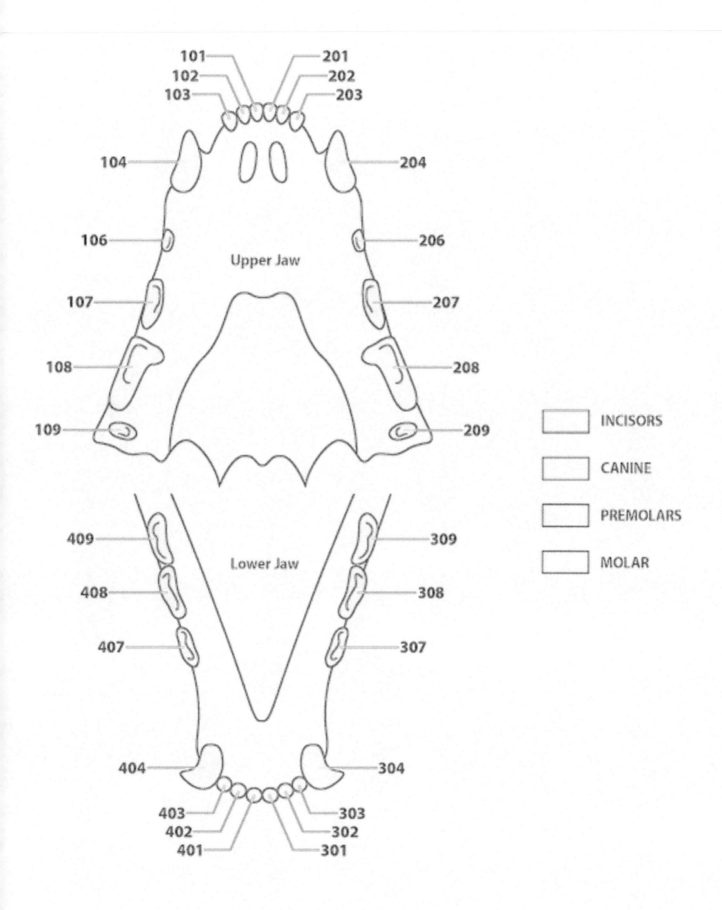

THE STAGES OF CARIES DEVELOPMENT

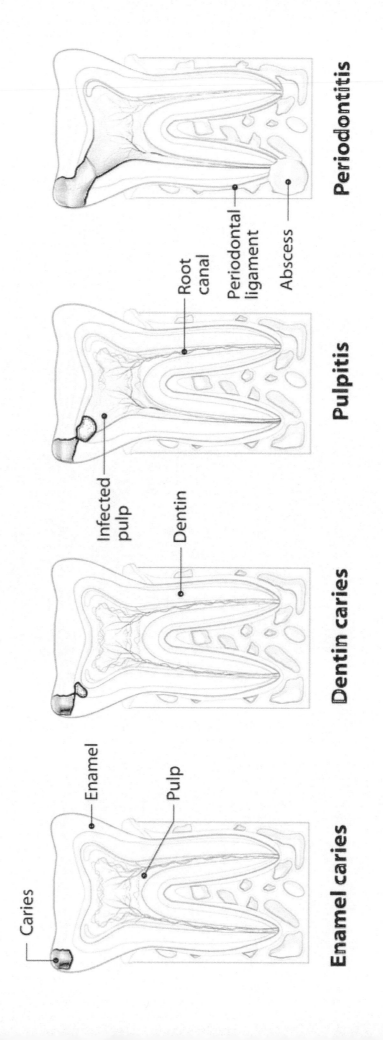

Caries

Enamel

Pulp

Enamel caries

Dentin caries

Infected pulp

Dentin

Root canal

Periodontal ligament

Abscess

Pulpitis

Periodontitis

Dental sketches. The structure of the teeth

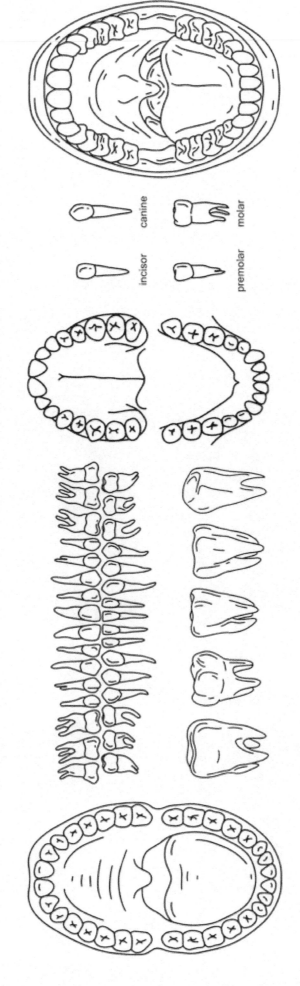

canine

molar

incisor

premolar

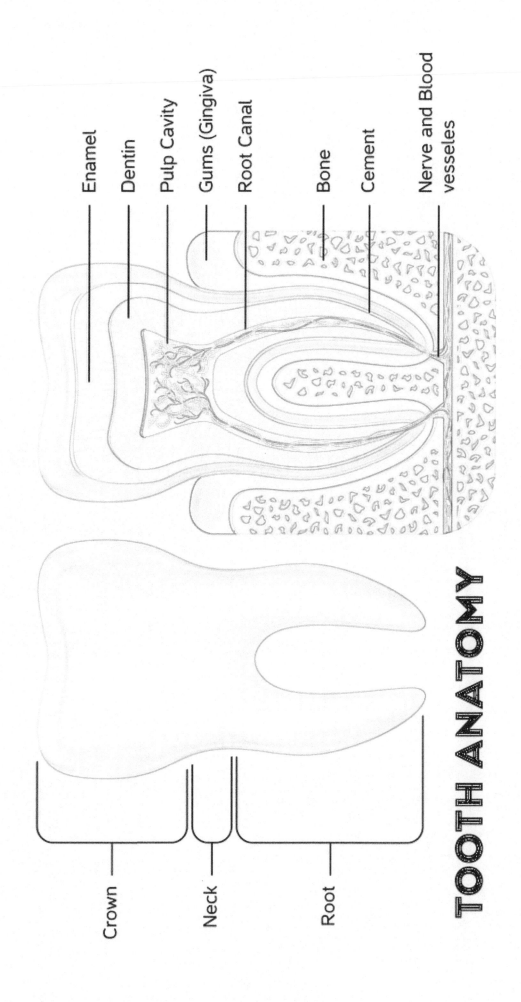

Enamel

Dentin

Pulp Cavity

Gums (Gingiva)

Root Canal

Bone

Cement

Nerve and Blood
vesseles

Crown

Neck

Root

TOOTH ANATOMY

TOOTH ANATOMY

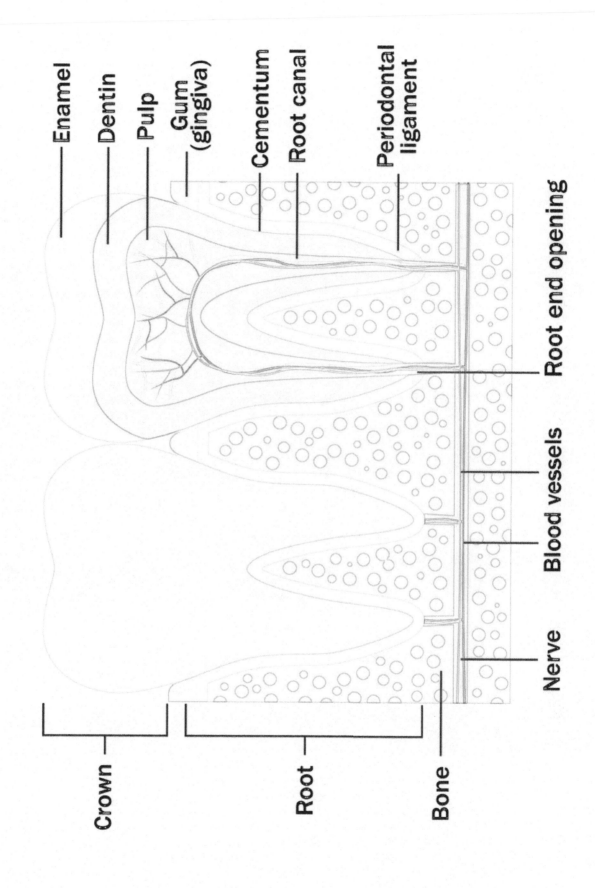

Enamel

Dentin

Pulp

Gum (gingiva)

Cementum

Root canal

Periodontal ligament

Root end opening

Blood vessels

Nerve

Crown

Root

Bone

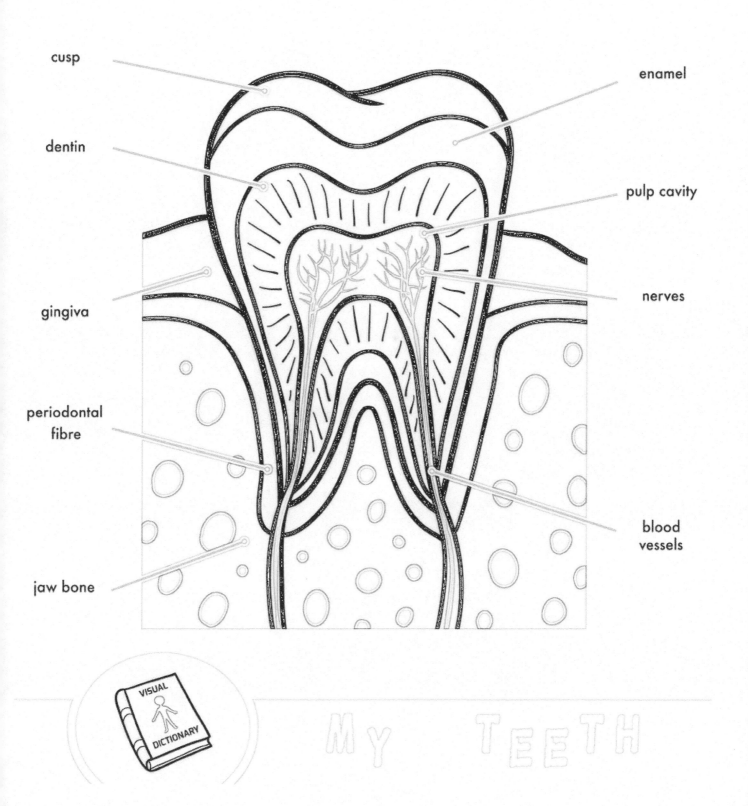

cusp

enamel

dentin

pulp cavity

gingiva

nerves

periodontal
fibre

blood
vessels

jaw bone

My Teeth

Dental anatomy

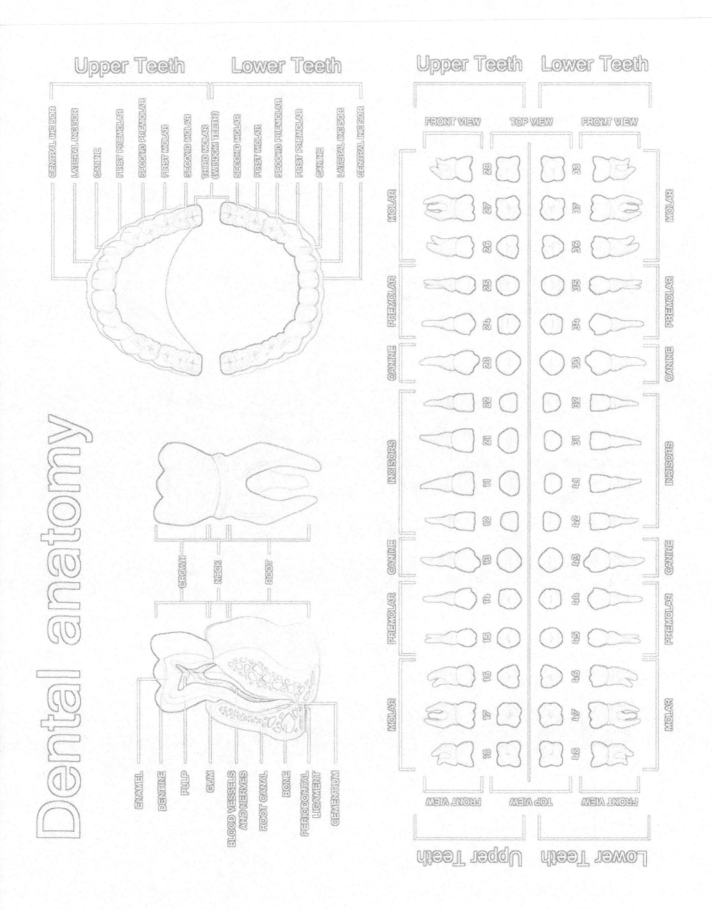

Root Canal Treatment

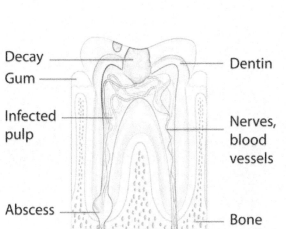

Decay
Gum
Infected pulp
Abscess
Dentin
Nerves, blood vessels
Bone

Infected tooth

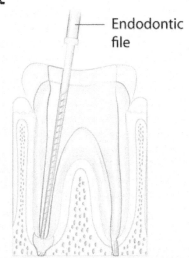

Opening

Opening made in tooth

Endodontic file

Infected tissue removed; Canals cleaned

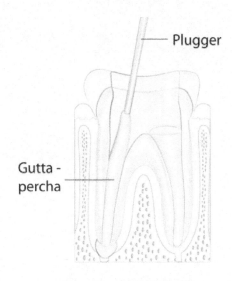

Plugger

Gutta - percha

Canals filled with a permanent material (gutta - percha)

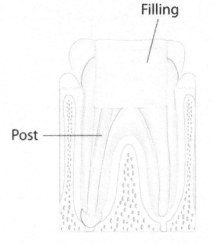

Filling

Post

Opening sealed with filling. In some cases, a post is inserted for extra support

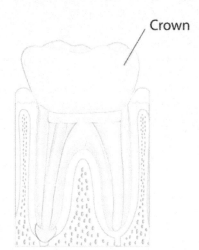

Crown

New crown cemented onto rebuilt tooth

TOOTH ANATOMY

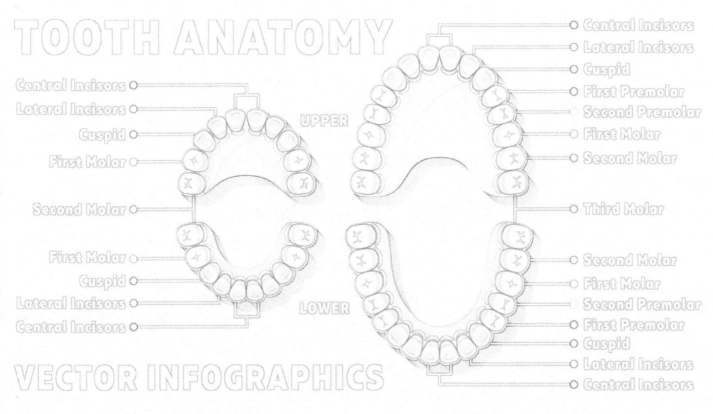

Central Incisors
Lateral Incisors
Cuspid
First Molar

Second Molar

First Molar
Cuspid
Lateral Incisors
Central Incisors

UPPER

LOWER

Central Incisors
Lateral Incisors
Cuspid
First Premolar
Second Premolar
First Molar
Second Molar

Third Molar

Second Molar
First Molar
Second Premolar
First Premolar
Cuspid
Lateral Incisors
Central Incisors

VECTOR INFOGRAPHICS

PRIMARY TEETH ERUPTION DATES

MONTHS			9		12	14		17			23			31
UPPER														
LOWER														
1		5		8	10		13		16			22	25	34

PERMANENT TEETH ERUPTION DATES

YEARS		6	8	10	12		17	
UPPER								
LOWER								
1		4	7	9	11	13		22

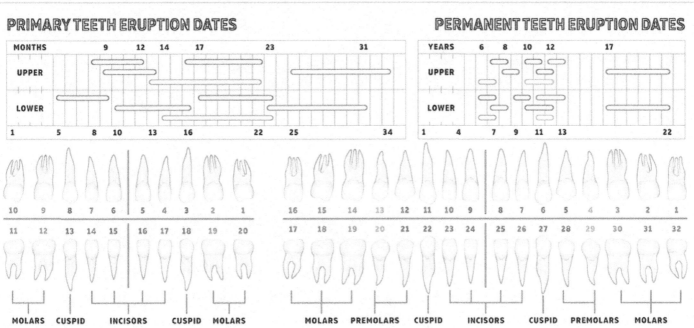

10	9	8	7	6	5	4	3	2	1

16	15	14	13	12	11	10	9	8	7	6	5	4	3	2	1

11	12	13	14	15	16	17	18	19	20

17	18	19	20	21	22	23	24	25	26	27	28	29	30	31	32

MOLARS CUSPID INCISORS CUSPID MOLARS

MOLARS PREMOLARS CUSPID INCISORS CUSPID PREMOLARS MOLARS

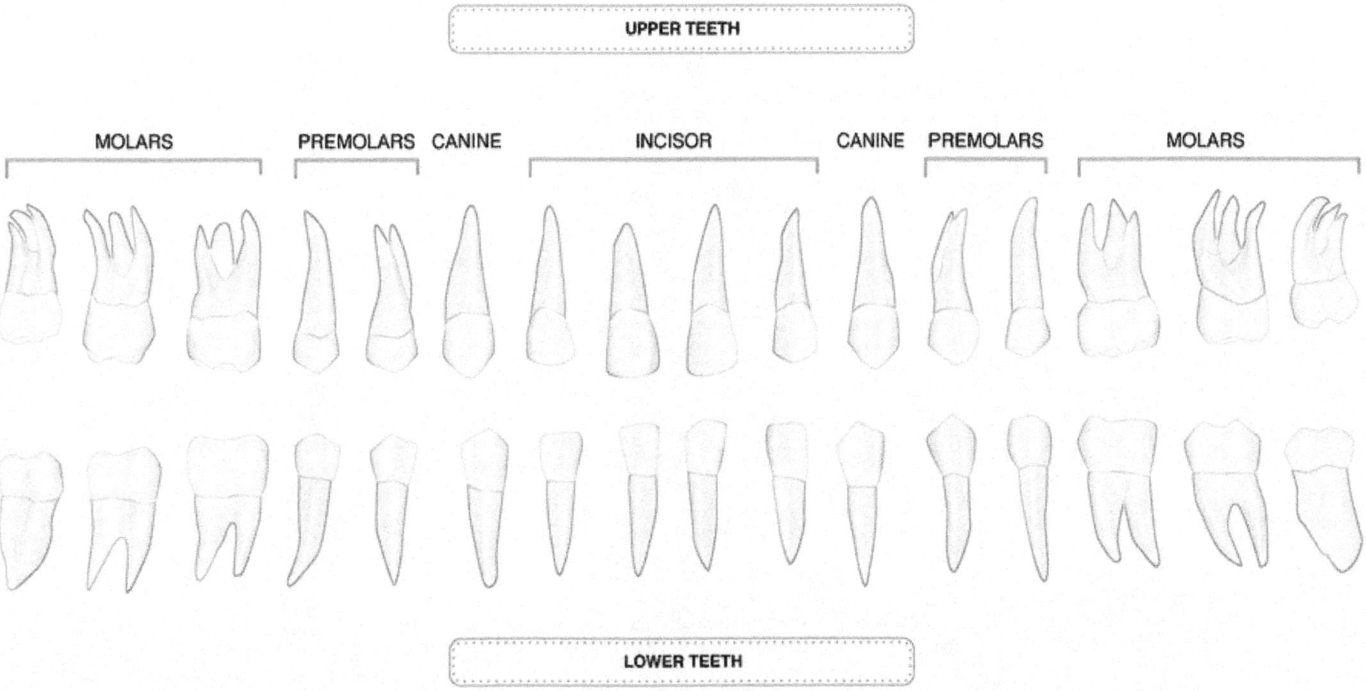
UPPER TEETH
MOLARS
PREMOLARS
CANINE
INCISOR
CANINE
PREMOLARS
MOLARS
LOWER TEETH

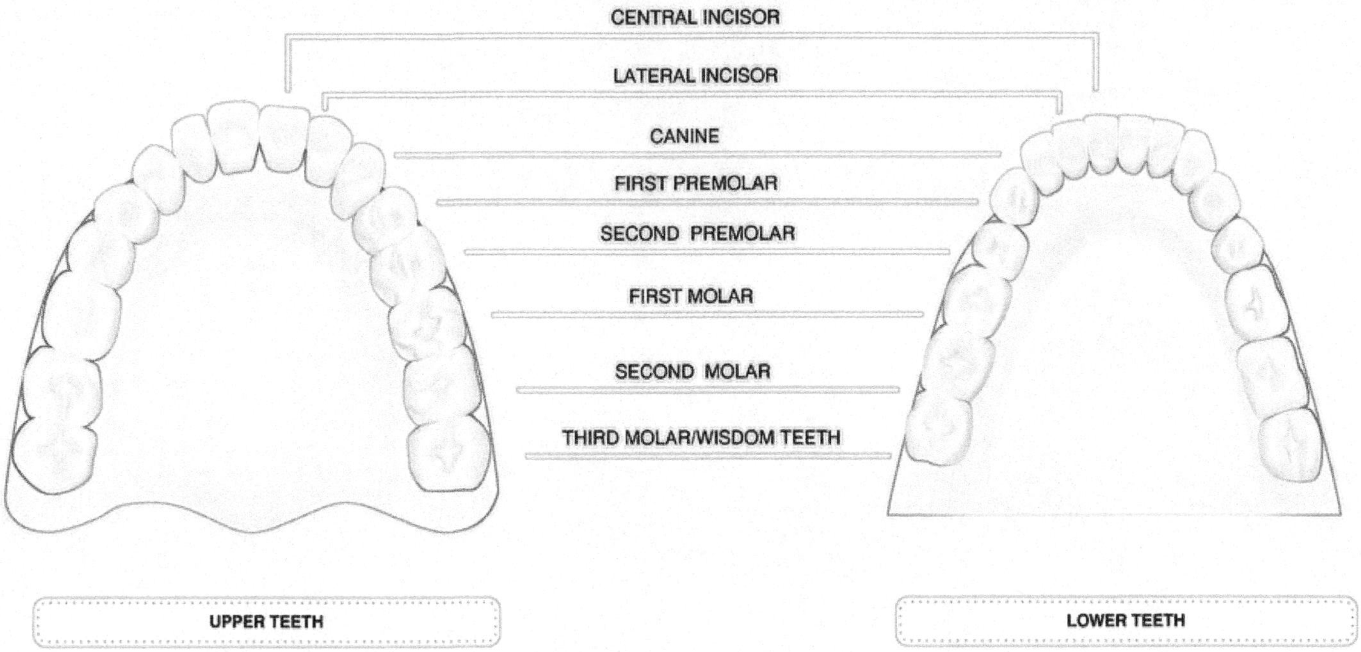
CENTRAL INCISOR
LATERAL INCISOR
CANINE
FIRST PREMOLAR
SECOND PREMOLAR
FIRST MOLAR
SECOND MOLAR
THIRD MOLAR/WISDOM TEETH
UPPER TEETH
LOWER TEETH

TOOTH
STRUCTURE

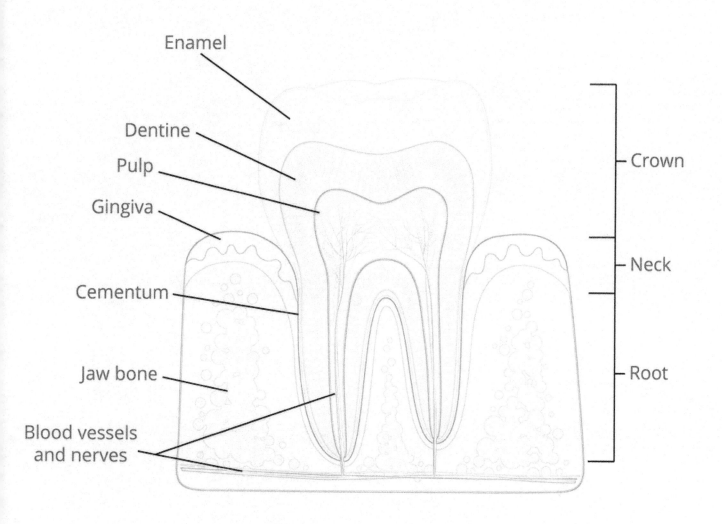

Enamel

Dentine

Pulp

Gingiva

Cementum

Jaw bone

Blood vessels
and nerves

Crown

Neck

Root

Tooth Anatomy

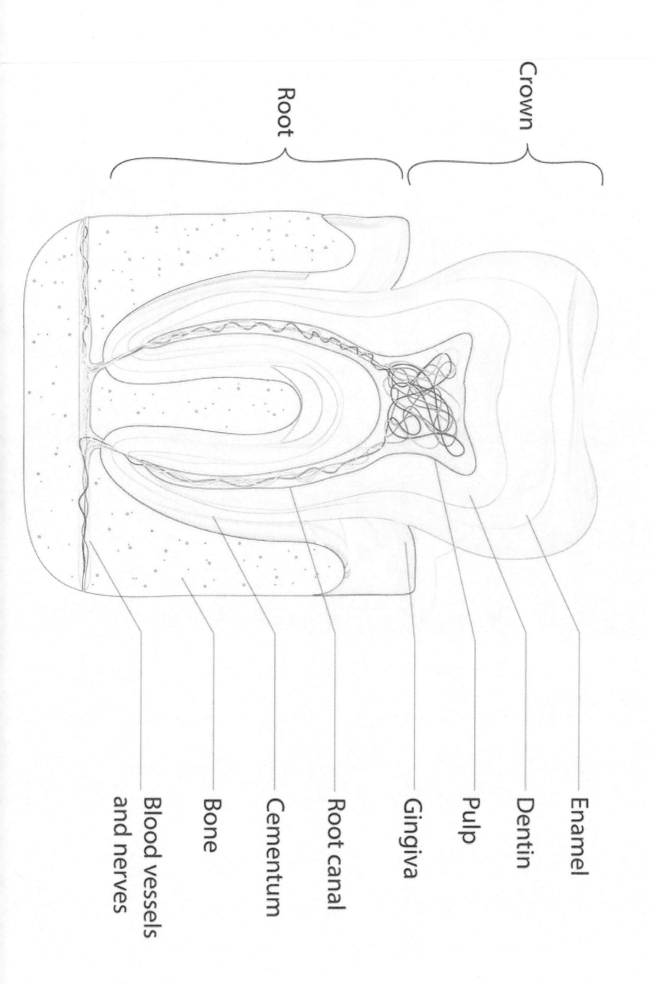

Crown

Root

Enamel

Dentin

Pulp

Gingiva

Root canal

Cementum

Bone

Blood vessels
and nerves

Dental Anatomy

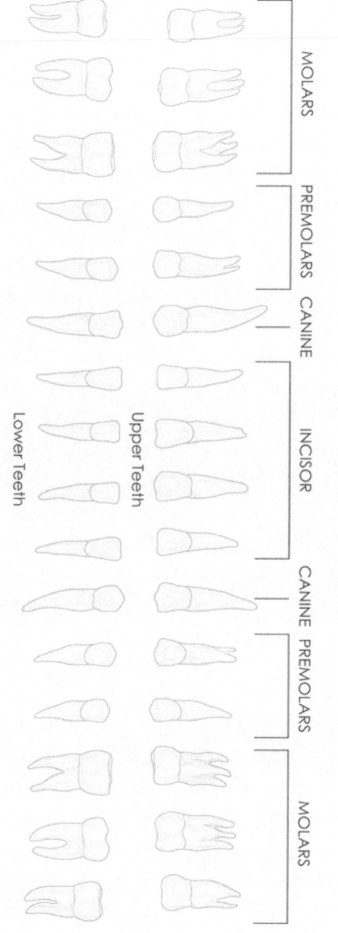

MOLARS

PREMOLARS

CANINE

INCISOR

CANINE

PREMOLARS

MOLARS

Upper Teeth

Lower Teeth

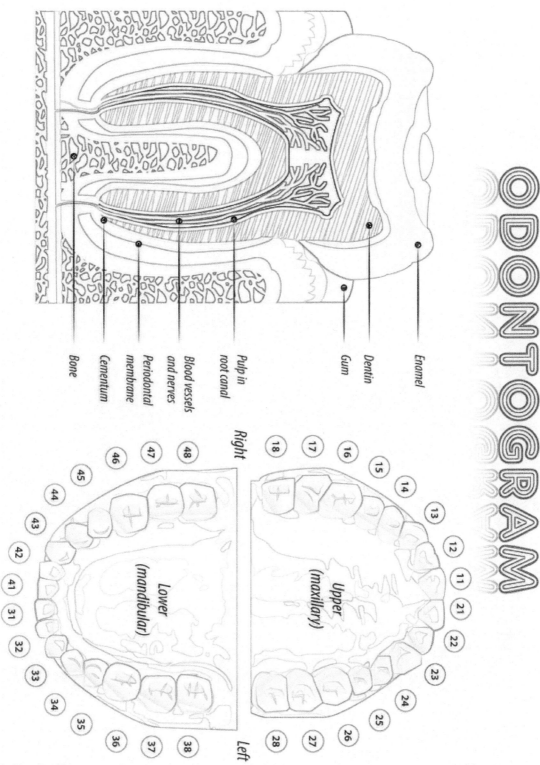

ODONTOGRAM

Crown

Root

Enamel

Gum

Dentin

Pulp in
root canal

Blood vessels
and nerves

Periodontal
membrane

Cementum

Bone

Right

Left

Upper
(maxillary)

Lower
(mandibular)

18
17
16
15
14
13
12
11
21
22
23
24
25
26
27
28

48
47
46
45
44
43
42
41
31
32
33
34
35
36
37
38

Incisors
Canines
Premolars
Molars

TYPES OF HUMAN PERMANENT TEETH

Dental formula:

$$(I\frac{}{}^2 C\frac{}{}^1 P\frac{}{}^2 M\frac{}{}^3)/(I_2 C_1 P_2 M_3) \times 2 = 32$$

Eruption (years)

Central incisor	7-8
Lateral incisor	8-9
Canine (cuspid)	11-12
First premolar (first bicuspid)	10-11
Second premolar (second bicuspid)	10-12
First molar	6-7
Second molar	12-13
Third molar (Wisdom tooth)	17-21

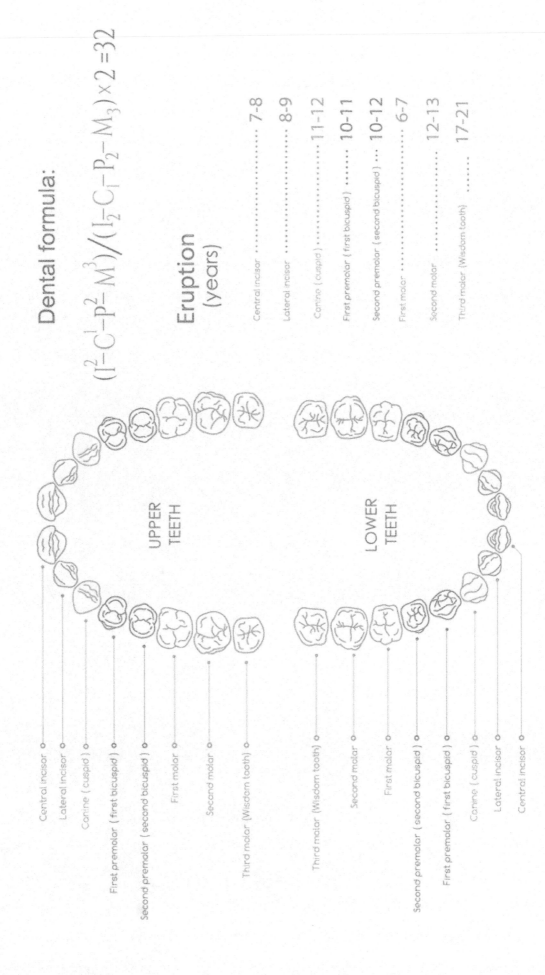

UPPER TEETH

- Central incisor
- Lateral incisor
- Canine (cuspid)
- First premolar (first bicuspid)
- Second premolar (second bicuspid)
- First molar
- Second molar
- Third molar (Wisdom tooth)

LOWER TEETH

- Third molar (Wisdom tooth)
- Second molar
- First molar
- Second premolar (second bicuspid)
- First premolar (first bicuspid)
- Canine (cuspid)
- Lateral incisor
- Central incisor

TOOTH ANATOMY

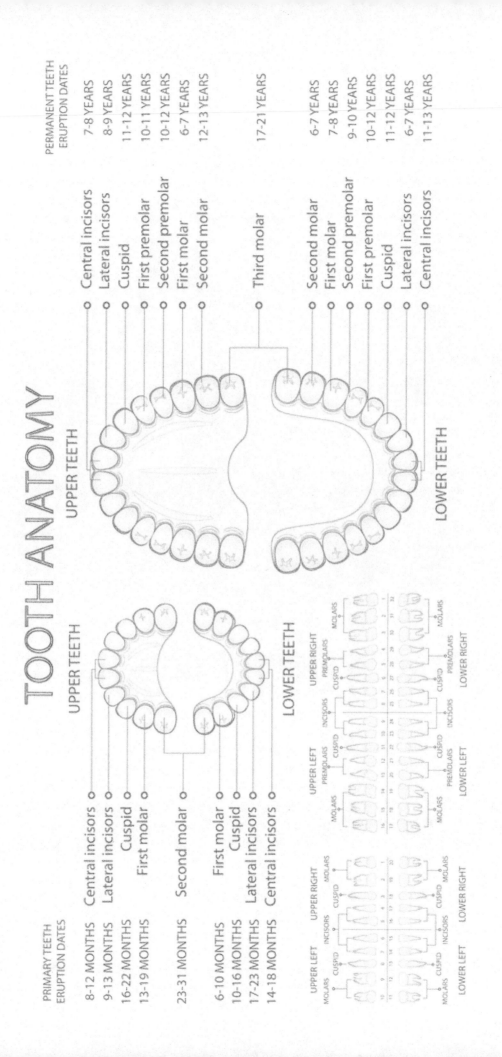

PERMANENT TEETH ERUPTION DATES

UPPER TEETH

Tooth	Eruption
Central incisors	7-8 YEARS
Lateral incisors	8-9 YEARS
Cuspid	11-12 YEARS
First premolar	10-11 YEARS
Second premolar	10-12 YEARS
First molar	6-7 YEARS
Second molar	12-13 YEARS
Third molar	17-21 YEARS

LOWER TEETH

Tooth	Eruption
Second molar	6-7 YEARS
First molar	7-8 YEARS
Second premolar	9-10 YEARS
First premolar	10-12 YEARS
Cuspid	11-12 YEARS
Lateral incisors	6-7 YEARS
Central incisors	11-13 YEARS

PRIMARY TEETH ERUPTION DATES

UPPER TEETH

Tooth	Eruption
Central incisors	8-12 MONTHS
Lateral incisors	9-13 MONTHS
Cuspid	16-22 MONTHS
First molar	13-19 MONTHS
Second molar	23-31 MONTHS

LOWER TEETH

Tooth	Eruption
First molar	6-10 MONTHS
Cuspid	10-16 MONTHS
Lateral incisors	17-23 MONTHS
Central incisors	14-18 MONTHS

Adult dental chart

Eruption (year)

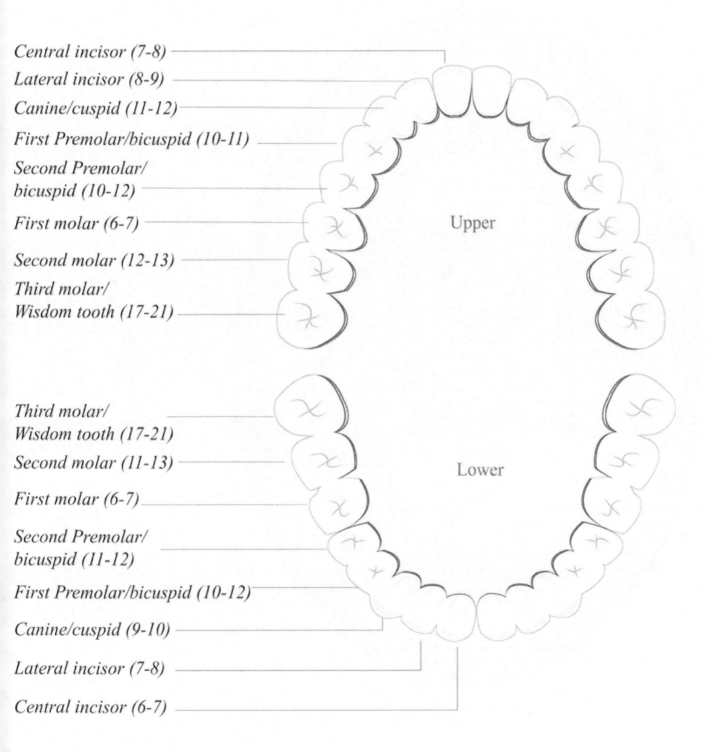

Central incisor (7-8)

Lateral incisor (8-9)

Canine/cuspid (11-12)

First Premolar/bicuspid (10-11)

Second Premolar/
bicuspid (10-12)

First molar (6-7)

Second molar (12-13)

Third molar/
Wisdom tooth (17-21)

Upper

Third molar/
Wisdom tooth (17-21)

Second molar (11-13)

First molar (6-7)

Second Premolar/
bicuspid (11-12)

First Premolar/bicuspid (10-12)

Canine/cuspid (9-10)

Lateral incisor (7-8)

Central incisor (6-7)

Lower

DENTAL INFOGRAPHICS

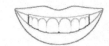

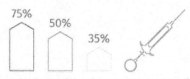

75%   50%   35%

Lorem ipsum dolor sitamet, consectetur adi
pisicing elit, sed do eiusmod tempor inci
didunt ut labore et dolore magna aliqua.

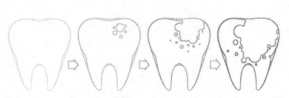

CARIES

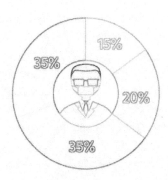

15%
35%
20%
35%

○ Lorem ipsum dolor sit amet,
consectetur adipisicing elit, sed
do eiusmod tempor incididunt
ut labore et dolore magna aliqua.

○ Nemo enim ipsam voluptatem
quia voluptas sit aspernatur aut
odit aut fugit, sed quia consequ
one voluptatem sequi nesvciunt.

○ Lorem ipsum dolor sit amet,
consectetur adipisicing elit, sed
do eiusmod tempor incididunt
ut labore et dolore magna aliqua.

○ Ut enim ad minim veniam, quis
nostrud exercitation ullamco
laboris nisi ut aliquip ex ea com
modo consequat.

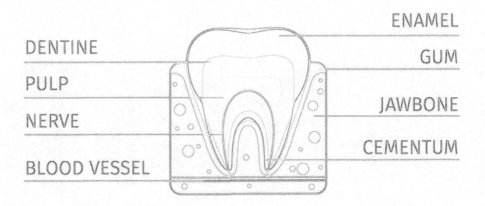

DENTINE   ENAMEL

PULP   GUM

NERVE   JAWBONE

BLOOD VESSEL   CEMENTUM

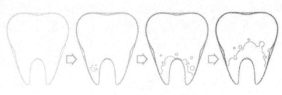

CALCULUS

70%

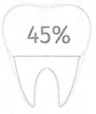

Lorem ipsum dolor sitamet, consectetur adi
pisicing elit, sed do eiusmod tempor inci
didunt ut labore et dolore magna aliqua.

45%

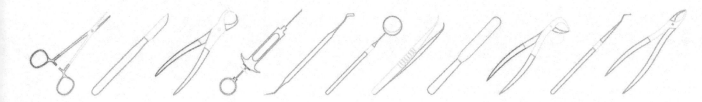

The stages of caries development

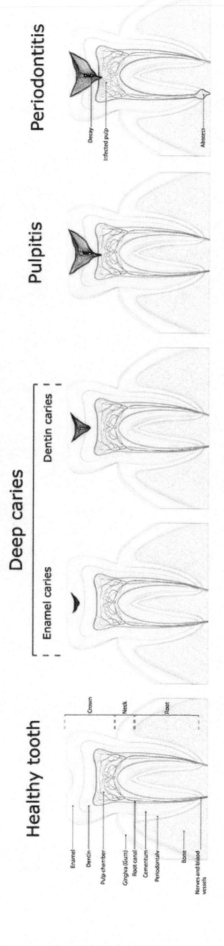

Healthy tooth

Deep caries

Enamel caries | Dentin caries

Pulpitis

Periodontitis

Enamel
Dentin
Pulp chamber
Gingiva (Gum)
Root canal
Cementum
Periodontium
Bone
Nerves and blood vessels

Crown
Neck
Root

Decay
Infected pulp
Abscess

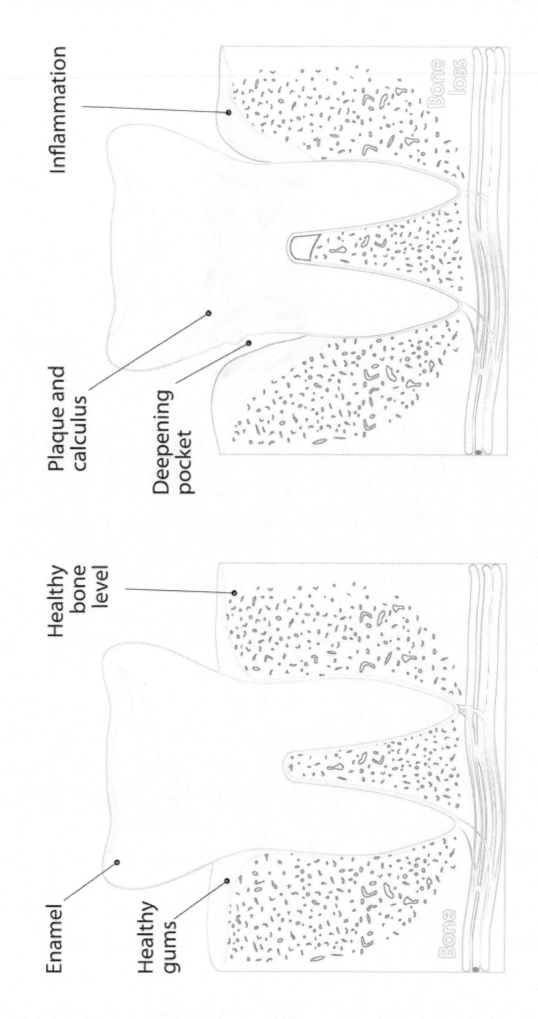

Periodontitis

Inflammation

Plaque and calculus

Deepening pocket

Bone loss

Normal tooth

Healthy bone level

Enamel

Healthy gums

Bone

Tooth anatomy

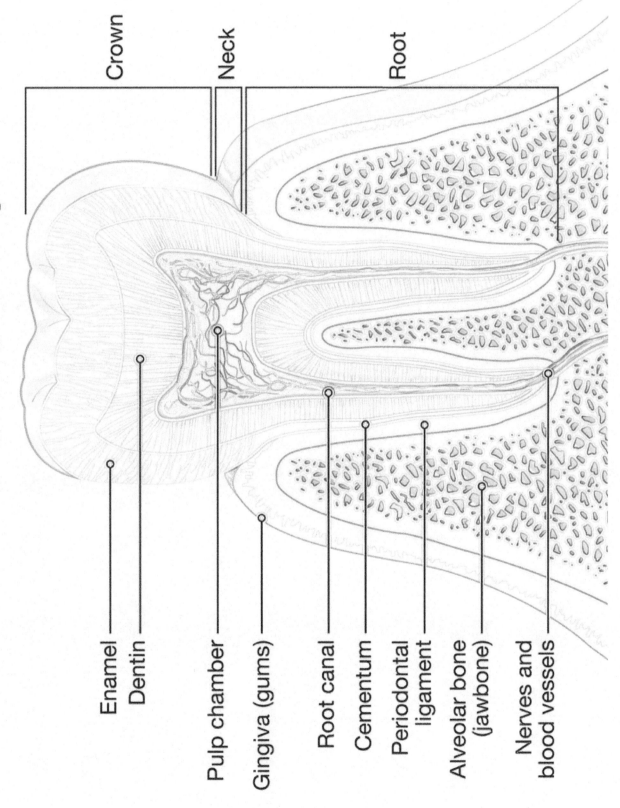

Crown

Neck

Root

Enamel

Dentin

Pulp chamber

Gingiva (gums)

Root canal

Cementum

Periodontal ligament

Alveolar bone (jawbone)

Nerves and blood vessels

Tooth (section of a molar)

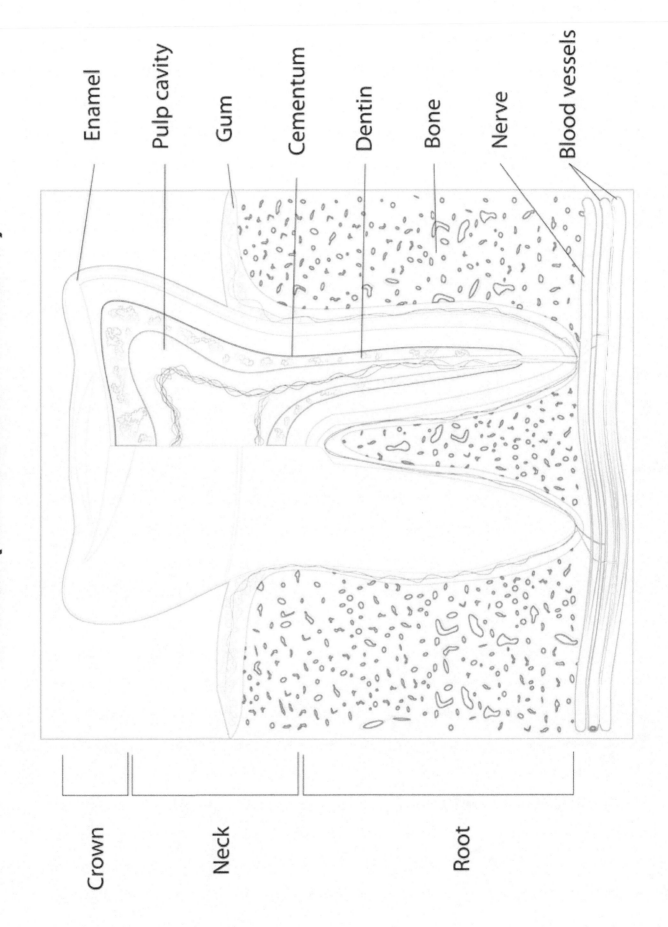

Enamel

Pulp cavity

Gum

Cementum

Dentin

Bone

Nerve

Blood vessels

Crown

Neck

Root

FORMS OF CARIES

I spot

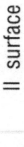

Lorem Ipsum is simply dummy text of the printing and typesetting industry. Lorem Ipsum has been the industry's standard dummy text ever since the 1500s

II surface

Lorem Ipsum is simply dummy text of the printing and typesetting industry. Lorem Ipsum has been the industry's standard dummy text ever since the 1500s

III average

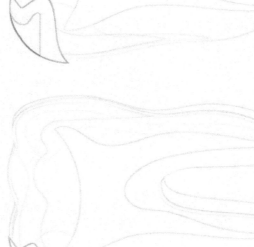

Lorem Ipsum is simply dummy text of the printing and typesetting industry. Lorem Ipsum has been the industry's standard dummy text ever since the 1500s

IV deep

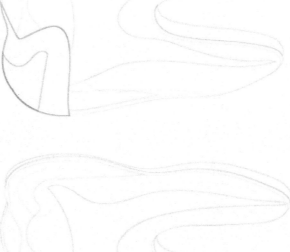

Lorem Ipsum is simply dummy text of the printing and typesetting industry. Lorem Ipsum has been the industry's standard dummy text ever since the 1500s

DENTAL BRIDGE

Bridge

Lorem ipsum dolor sit amet, consectetur adipiscing elit, sed do eiusmod tempor incididunt ut labore et dolore magna aliqua. Ut enim ad minim veniam, quis nostrud exercitation ullamco laboris nisi ut aliquip ex ea commodo consequat.

Crown

Lorem ipsum dolor sit amet, consectetur adipiscing elit, sed do eiusmod tempor incididunt ut labore et dolore magna aliqua. Ut enim ad minim veniam, quis nostrud exercitation ullamco laboris nisi ut aliquip ex ea commodo consequat.

Cementum

Lorem ipsum dolor sit amet, consectetur adipiscing elit, sed do eiusmod tempor incididunt ut labore et dolore magna aliqua. Ut enim ad minim veniam, quis nostrud exercitation ullamco laboris nisi ut aliquip ex ea commodo consequat.

Pontic

Crown

Gingiva

Lorem ipsum dolor sit amet, consectetur adipiscing elit, sed do eiusmod tempor incididunt ut labore et dolore magna aliqua. Ut enim ad minim veniam, quis nostrud exercitation ullamco laboris nisi ut aliquip ex ea commodo consequat.

Periodontal ligament

Lorem ipsum dolor sit amet, consectetur adipiscing elit, sed do eiusmod tempor incididunt ut labore et dolore magna aliqua. Ut enim ad minim veniam, quis nostrud exercitation ullamco laboris nisi ut aliquip ex ea commodo consequat.

Jaw bone

Lorem ipsum dolor sit amet, consectetur adipiscing elit, sed do eiusmod tempor incididunt ut labore et dolore magna aliqua. Ut enim ad minim veniam, quis nostrud exercitation ullamco laboris nisi ut aliquip ex ea commodo consequat.

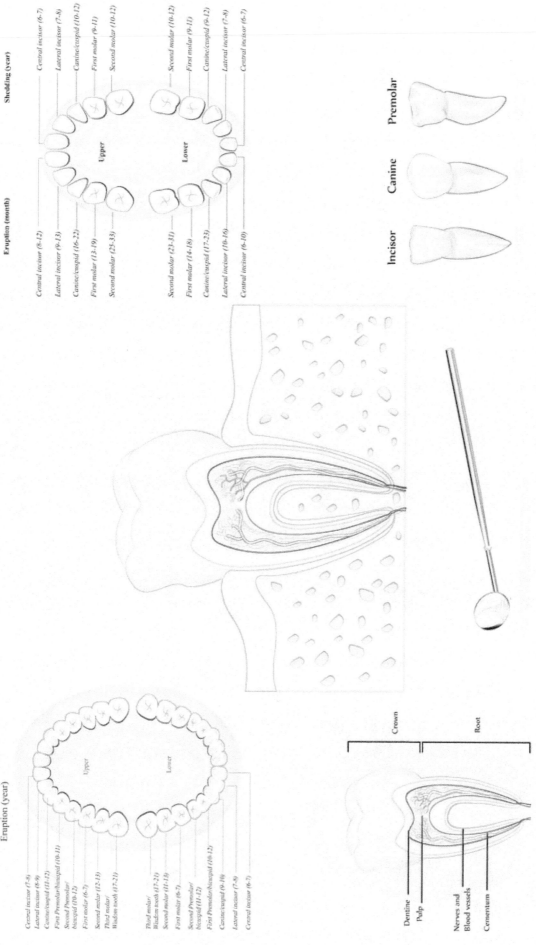

Tooth Anatomy

Children dental chart

Shedding (year)
- Central incisor (6-7)
- Lateral incisor (7-8)
- Canine/cuspid (10-12)
- First molar (9-11)
- Second molar (10-12)
- Second molar (10-12)
- First molar (9-11)
- Canine/cuspid (10-12)
- Lateral incisor (7-8)
- Central incisor (6-7)

Upper / Lower

Eruption (month)
- Central incisor (8-12)
- Lateral incisor (9-13)
- Canine/cuspid (16-22)
- First molar (13-19)
- Second molar (25-33)
- Second molar (23-31)
- First molar (14-18)
- Canine/cuspid (17-23)
- Lateral incisor (10-16)
- Central incisor (6-10)

Adult dental chart

Eruption (year)
- Central incisor (7-8)
- Lateral incisor (8-9)
- Canine/cuspid (11-12)
- First Premolar/bicuspid (10-11)
- Second Premolar/bicuspid (10-12)
- First molar (6-7)
- Second molar (12-13)
- Third molar/Wisdom tooth (17-21)
- Third molar/Wisdom tooth (17-21)
- Second molar (11-13)
- First molar (6-7)
- Second Premolar/bicuspid (10-12)
- First Premolar/bicuspid (10-12)
- Canine/cuspid (9-10)
- Lateral incisor (7-8)
- Central incisor (6-7)

Upper / Lower

Incisor　　Canine　　Premolar

Crown

Root

- Dentine
- Pulp
- Nerves and Blood vessels
- Cementum

ADULT DENTAL ANATOMY

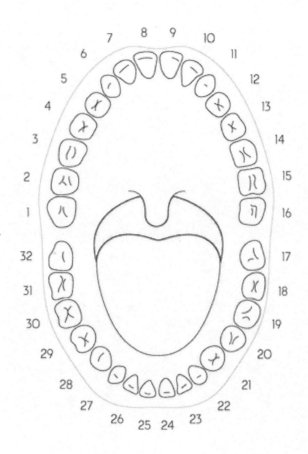

UPPER RIGHT:

1. 3rd Molar / Wisdom tooth
2. 2nd Molar
3. 1st Molar
4. 2nd Premolar
5. 1st Premolar
6. Cuspid
7. Lateral Incisors
8. Central Incisors

LOWER RIGHT:

25. Central Incisors
26. Lateral Incisors
27. Cuspid
28. 1st Premolar
29. 2nd Premolar
30. 1st Molar
31. 2nd Molar
32. 3rd Molar / Wisdom tooth

UPPER LEFT:

9. Central Incisors
10. Lateral Incisors
11. Cuspid
12. 1st Premolar
13. 2nd Premolar
14. 1st Molar
15. 2nd Molar
16. 3rd Molar / Wisdom tooth

LOWER LEFT:

17. 3rd Molar / Wisdom tooth
18. 2nd Molar
19. 1st Molar
20. 2nd Premolar
21. 1st Premolar
22. Cuspid
23. Lateral Incisors
24. Central Incisors

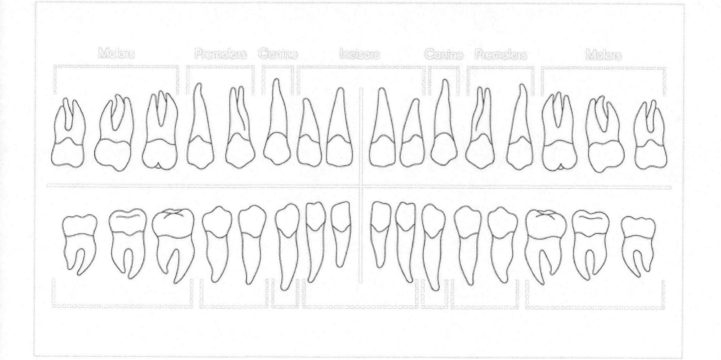

Molars   Premolars   Canine   Incisors   Canine   Premolars   Molars

Permanent Teeth

Incisors

Canines

Premolars

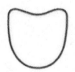

Molars

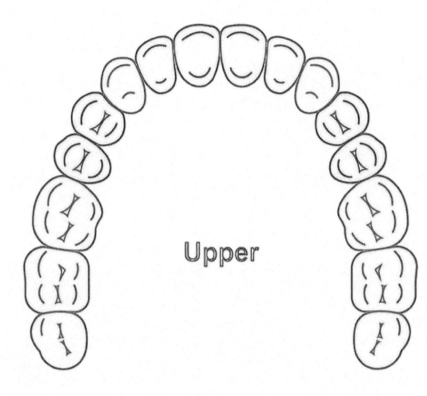

Upper

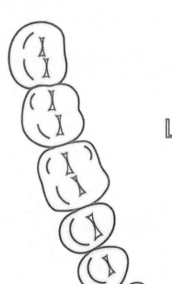
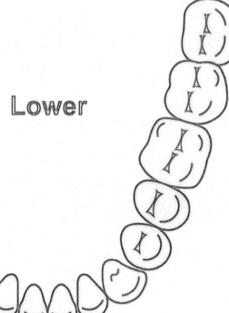

Lower

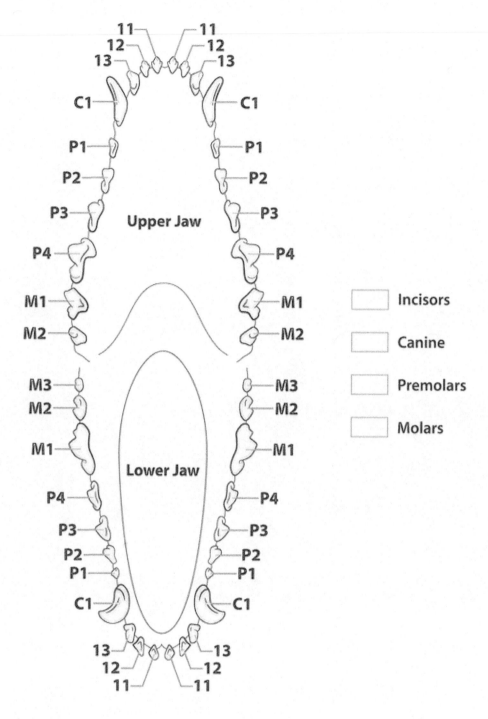

I1
I2
I3
C1
P1
P2
P3
P4
M1
M2

Upper Jaw

Incisors

Canine

Premolars

Molars

M3
M2
M1
P4
P3
P2
P1
C1

Lower Jaw

I3
I2
I1

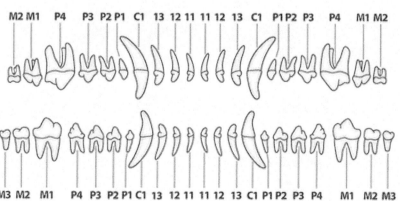

M2 M1 P4 P3 P2 P1 C1 I3 I2 I1 I1 I2 I3 C1 P1 P2 P3 P4 M1 M2

M3 M2 M1 P4 P3 P2 P1 C1 I3 I2 I1 I1 I2 I3 C1 P1 P2 P3 P4 M1 M2 M3

Adult dental chart

Eruption (year)

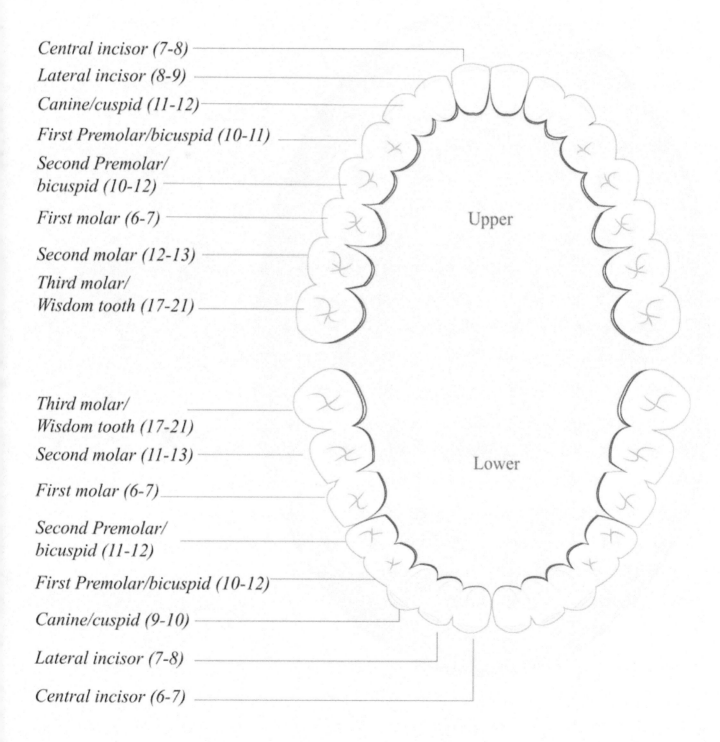

Central incisor (7-8)

Lateral incisor (8-9)

Canine/cuspid (11-12)

First Premolar/bicuspid (10-11)

Second Premolar/
bicuspid (10-12)

First molar (6-7)

Second molar (12-13)

Third molar/
Wisdom tooth (17-21)

Upper

Third molar/
Wisdom tooth (17-21)

Second molar (11-13)

First molar (6-7)

Second Premolar/
bicuspid (11-12)

First Premolar/bicuspid (10-12)

Canine/cuspid (9-10)

Lateral incisor (7-8)

Central incisor (6-7)

Lower

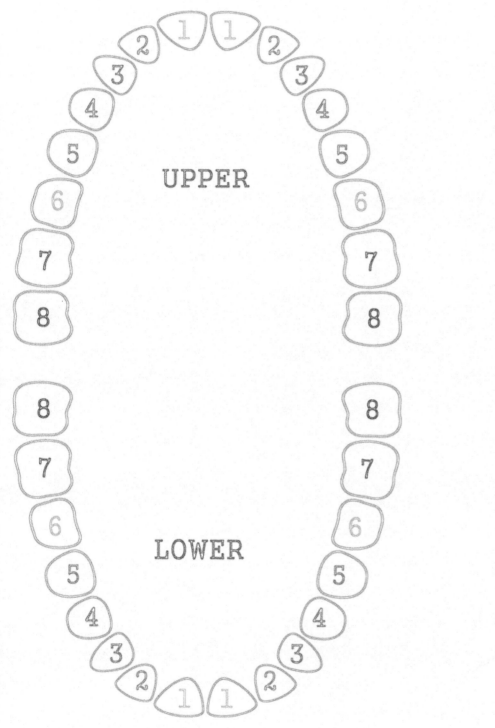

UPPER

1	7-8	YEARS
2	8-9	YEARS
3	11-12	YEARS
4	10-11	YEARS
5	10-12	YEARS
6	6-7	YEARS
7	12-13	YEARS
8	17-21	YERAS

LOWER

1	6-7	YEARS
2	7-8	YEARS
3	9-10	YEARS
4	10-12	YEARS
5	11-12	YEARS
6	6-7	YEARS
7	11-13	YEARS
8	17-21	YERAS

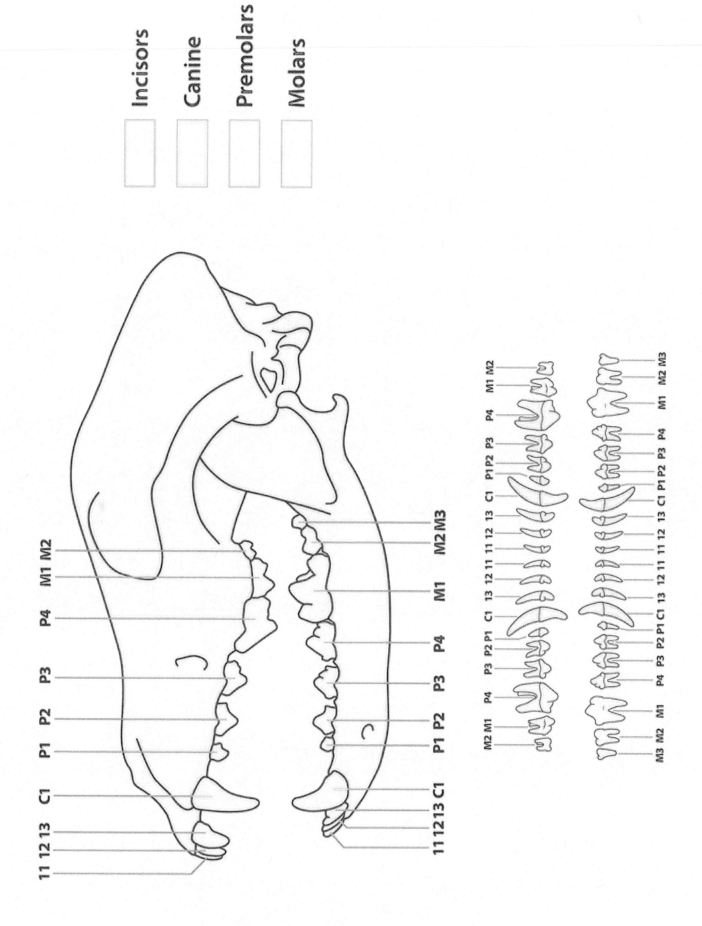

Incisors

Canine

Premolars

Molars

I1 I2 I3 C1 P1 P2 P3 P4 M1 M2

I1 I2 I3 C1 P1 P2 P3 P4 M1 M2 M3

Dental problems

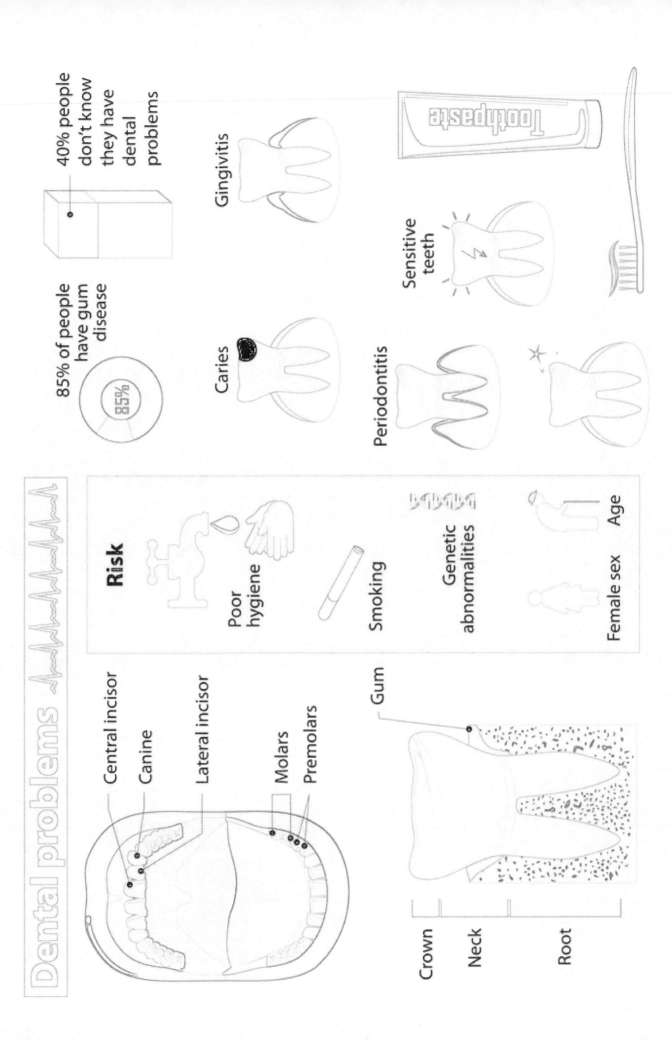

40% people don't know they have dental problems

85% of people have gum disease

85%

Gingivitis

Caries

Sensitive teeth

Periodontitis

Toothpaste

Risk

Poor hygiene

Smoking

Genetic abnormalities

Female sex

Age

Central incisor

Canine

Lateral incisor

Molars

Premolars

Gum

Crown

Neck

Root

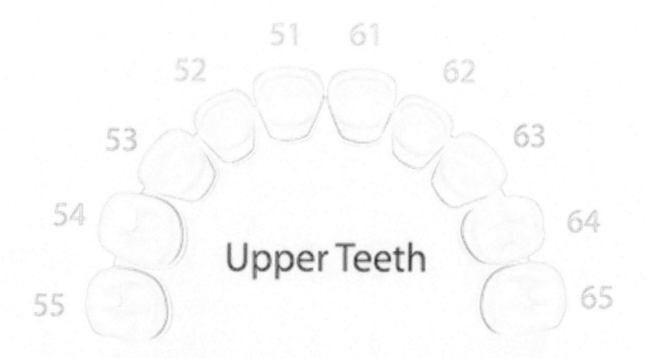

51 61

52 62

53 63

54 64

55 65

Upper Teeth

Deciduous Dentition

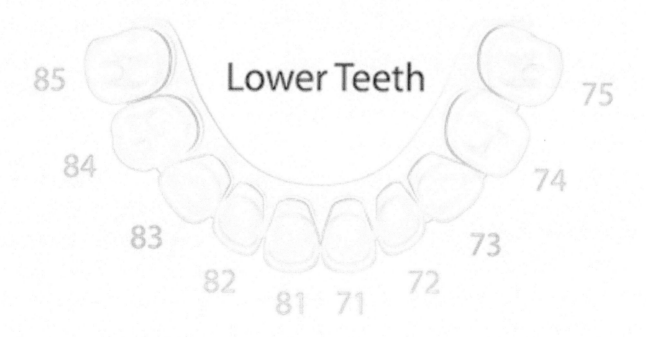

Lower Teeth

85 75

84 74

83 73

82 72

81 71

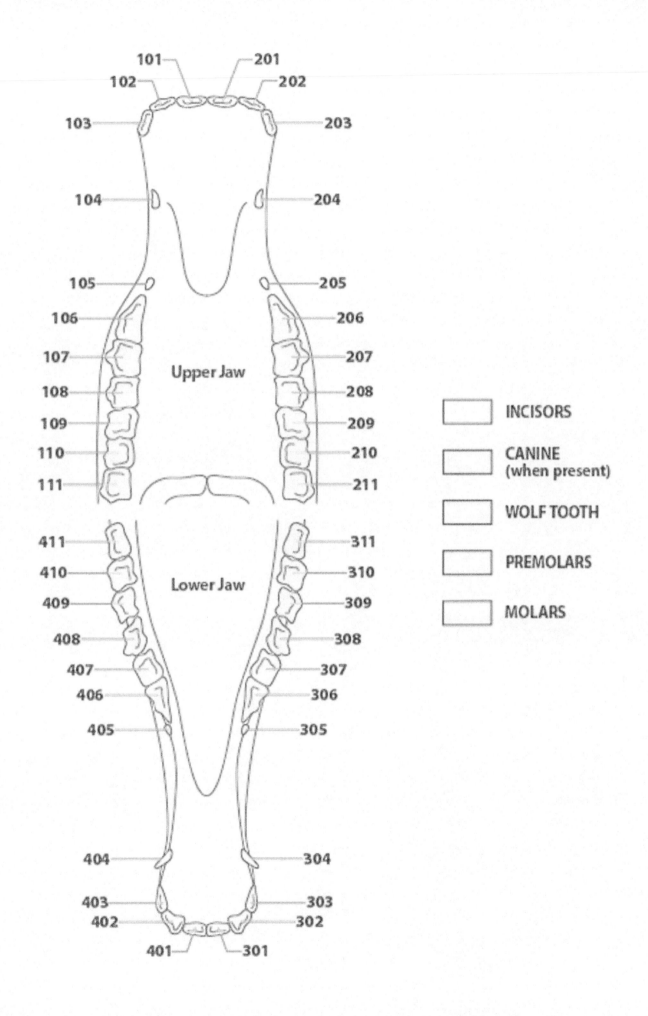

101		201
102		202
103		203
104		204
105		205
106		206
107		207
108	Upper Jaw	208
109		209
110		210
111		211

411		311
410	Lower Jaw	310
409		309
408		308
407		307
406		306
405		305
404		304
403		303
402		302
401	301	

INCISORS

CANINE
(when present)

WOLF TOOTH

PREMOLARS

MOLARS

TOOTH ANATOMY
VECTOR INFOGRAPHIC

UPPER TEETH

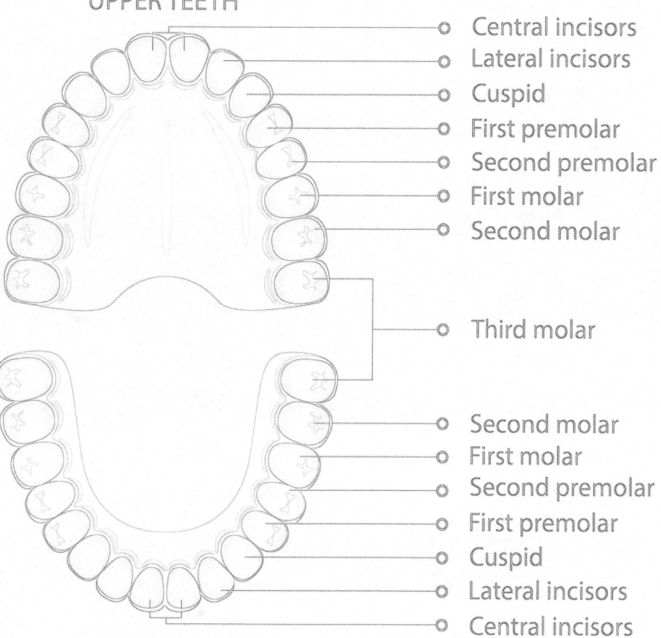

- Central incisors
- Lateral incisors
- Cuspid
- First premolar
- Second premolar
- First molar
- Second molar

- Third molar

- Second molar
- First molar
- Second premolar
- First premolar
- Cuspid
- Lateral incisors
- Central incisors

LOWER TEETH

DENTAL NUMBERING SYSTEMS

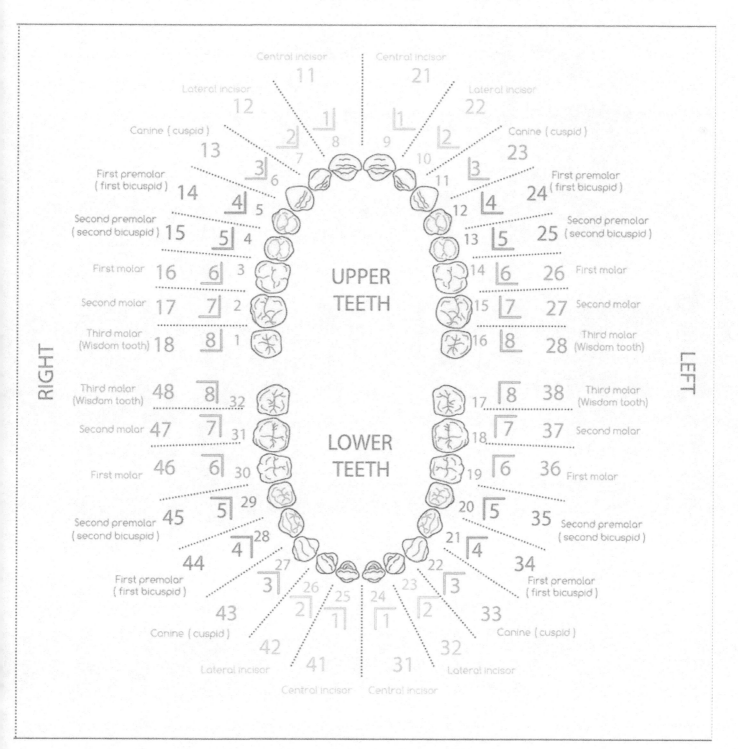

RIGHT

LEFT

UPPER TEETH

LOWER TEETH

Central incisor — 11 / 21 — Central incisor
Lateral incisor — 12 / 22 — Lateral incisor
Canine (cuspid) — 13 / 23 — Canine (cuspid)
First premolar (first bicuspid) — 14 / 24 — First premolar (first bicuspid)
Second premolar (second bicuspid) — 15 / 25 — Second premolar (second bicuspid)
First molar — 16 / 26 — First molar
Second molar — 17 / 27 — Second molar
Third molar (Wisdom tooth) — 18 / 28 — Third molar (Wisdom tooth)

Third molar (Wisdom tooth) — 48 / 38 — Third molar (Wisdom tooth)
Second molar — 47 / 37 — Second molar
First molar — 46 / 36 — First molar
Second premolar (second bicuspid) — 45 / 35 — Second premolar (second bicuspid)
First premolar (first bicuspid) — 44 / 34 — First premolar (first bicuspid)
Canine (cuspid) — 43 / 33 — Canine (cuspid)
Lateral incisor — 42 / 32 — Lateral incisor
Central incisor — 41 / 31 — Central incisor

PERMANENT TEETH

Dental implant with crown

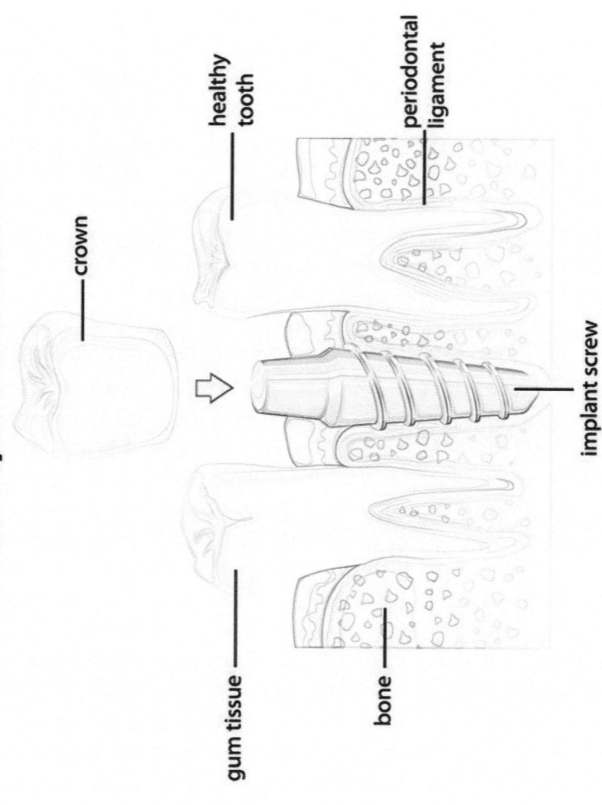

crown

healthy tooth

periodontal ligament

implant screw

gum tissue

bone

THANKS FOR BEING
WITH US
I HOPE WE ARE I
IMPROVED
DENTAL ANATOMY
EXPERIENCE

SO DON'T FORGET TO
CHECK OUT OTHERS PRODUCTS ON OUR AUTHOR